# A Practical Approach to Pediatric Gastroenterology

# A Practical Approach to Pediatric Gastroenterology

**Joseph Levy, M.D., F.A.A.P.**

Associate Clinical Professor of Pediatrics
Columbia University College of Physicians and Surgeons
Associate Physician
Columbia Presbyterian Medical Center
Director, Clinical Gastroenterology Service
Division of Pediatric Gastroenterology and Nutrition
Babies Hospital
New York, New York

YEAR BOOK MEDICAL PUBLISHERS, INC.
CHICAGO • LONDON • BOCA RATON

1 2 3 4 5 6 7 8 9 0 R Y 91 90 89 88 87

**Library of Congress Cataloging-in-Publication Data**

Levy, Joseph, 1946-
  A practical approach to pediatric gastroenterology.

  Includes bibliographies and index.
  1. Pediatric gastroenterology. I. Title.
[DNLM: 1. Gastrointestinal Diseases--in infancy &
childhood. WS 310 L668p]
RJ446.L48   1988      618.92'33      87-15978
ISBN 0-8151-5419-4

Sponsoring Editor: Stephany S. Scott
Manager, Copyediting Services: Frances M. Perveiler
Copyeditor: Francis A. Byrne
Production Manager, Text and Reference/Periodicals: Etta Worthington
Proofroom Supervisor: Shirley E. Taylor

*To my parents, Clemen and Alberto, for their love and support through the years.*

*To my wife, Valery, and our children, Nomi and Berti, who put up with the long hours, always encouraging, understanding, and full of compassion for my patients and their families.*

# Foreword

Pediatric gastroenterology has come of age but it is still a young specialty. Beginnings can be traced back to the past 20 years and the pioneers are still around. Dr. Levy is a distinguished member of the second generation of pediatric gastroenterology. His experience as a caregiver and a teacher to medical students, interns, residents, and pediatric GI trainees at one of the most prestigious medical schools has inspired this concise and well written text.

The format of the book is problem-oriented in the interest of practicality and immediate usefulness. Its aim is to bridge the gap between standard pediatric gastroenterology textbooks and the cursory discussion of gastrointestinal, pancreatic, and hepatic problems found in most general pediatric books. Dr. Levy offers precious bedside tips and "pearls" while guiding the reader through the 18 chapters. Although often synoptic, the approach is applied and stresses the message of collecting and interpreting clinical data.

This book will be a useful guide for housestaff, family physicians, and pediatricians. It should also prove helpful to pediatric gastroenterologists endeavoring to improve the "take-home pay" of their teaching.

CLAUDE C. ROY, M.D.
PROFESSOR OF PEDIATRICS
HOSPITAL SAINT-JUSTINE
MONTREAL, QUEBEC, CANADA

# Introduction

This manual was written with the practitioner in mind. It is meant to be a companion, an abbreviated refresher course on certain aspects of pediatric gastroenterology frequently encountered in the office. I have tried to include enough background basic information to offer a sensible approach to the diagnosis and management of the most common clinical entities.

The dialogue between the general practitioner and the specialist should be beneficial to both. This communication is at its best when there is an awareness of their respective strengths. When to refer and when to manage the patient with an intestinal dysfunction is an important decision made daily by the busy practitioner.

It is hoped that with the information provided in this book, a more realistic picture of the field of pediatric gastroenterology will emerge with a better sense of the great advances being made.

Pediatric gastroenterology has indeed grown into a full-fledged specialty in the past decade. Important information has been gathered on the mechanisms of disease and newer methodologies promise to maintain the momentum for years to come. For the pediatrician in practice, the task of keeping up with the developments in this field is becoming progressively more difficult. Exposure to periodicals and journals dealing specifically with pediatric gastrointestinal and nutritional problems is limited and the gap will only continue to widen.

Significant changes are taking place in the way certain diseases are understood and managed. For example, progress in intestinal physiology allows us to describe in great detail important functions such as fluid and electrolyte homeostasis in the gut. Elucidation of the serological changes in infectious hepatitis has revolutionized the way we approach the diagnosis of acute jaundice. New imaging modalities, more invasive methods of investigation and more specific pharmacologic interventions are resulting in faster and more precise diagnosis and an improved outlook for many patients.

Textbooks of pediatric gastroenterology cover the field in great detail but are generally aimed at the specialist who is often interested and needs more extensive and critical analysis of the original references. Monographs and proceedings of clinical and research symposia have also proliferated in the past years, expanding further the scope of new information in this field.

For the busy practitioner, a concise and practical source of information is still needed. The challenge of producing such a guide and reference book was undertaken because of the perceived need to complement the continuing education of the physician and the positive effect that such updating would have on their approach to gastrointestinal disease.

If the pages of this book become discolored by frequent use and the information helps sharpen the skills of the practitioner, my goal will be fulfilled. Pediatric gastroenterology is an exciting field and its accomplishments should extend to the broadest base of health care providers.

I would like to take this opportunity to express my appreciation to all my co-workers and colleagues for their trust, suggestions, and the constant stimulation that makes academic practice such a challenging and exciting way of life. A special mention is due to my friend and mentor, Dr. Felipe Duran, who shared his love of science and the importance of compassion in the practice of medicine. To Dr. Walter Berdon, my thanks for his guidance, his inexhaustable inquisitiveness, and all those wonderful sailing escapades. Finally, my gratitude to Neal Bregman for always being there and for sharing the good things in life.

JOSEPH LEVY, M.D.

# Contents

# Vomiting and Gastroesophageal Reflux

Various forms of regurgitation occur frequently during infancy. In its most benign form, the baby "spits up" or has "wet burps," while in its more serious expression, the degree of vomiting results in compromised caloric intake and metabolic imbalance.

Generally speaking, the term gastroesophageal reflux (GER) is used to describe the unprovoked passage of gastric contents into the esophagus. In most cases, this is equivalent to acid/pepsin reflux, but bilious constituents might also be present ("alkaline reflux"), a result of retroperistalsis and duodenogastric reflux (Fig 1–1).

Much has been learned about the mechanisms determining the competence of the physiologic and anatomical barriers between the stomach and the esophagus. As new modalities of investigation are developed, these concepts change and become progressively more complex.

## ANATOMICAL AND PHYSIOLOGIC CONSIDERATIONS

The entrance of the esophagus into the abdominal cavity takes place between the crura of the diaphragm. A pinchcock mechanism provides a degree of angulation (angle of entrance), which helps in the closure of the lower esophageal sphincter (LES). The LES is not a true sphincter, but rather a group of muscle fibers from the esophagus and the stomach interlaced and strengthened by one

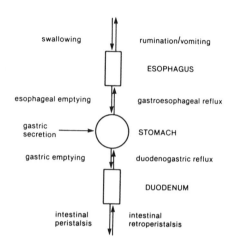

**FIG 1-1.**
The manifestations of abnormal swallowing, esophageal motility, and gastric emptying include rumination, gastroesophageal reflux, and duodenogastric reflux. (From Castell DO, Wu WC, Ott DJ (eds): *Gastroesophageal Reflux Disease: Pathogenesis, Diagnosis, Therapy.* Mount Kisco, New York, Futura Publishing Co, 1985. Used by permission.)

another under neurogenic, myogenic, and hormonal controls as depicted in Figure 1-2.

Increased intra-abdominal pressure will, under ideal circumstances, increase the pressure of closure of the LES, provided there are no abnormalities resulting in GE reflux. The lower esophageal sphincter can be detected by manometry, and its position is usually 3 cm to 5 cm above the junction of the esophagus and the stomach, unless a hiatal hernia is present, in which case it can be at any level in the mediastinum. The anatomical landmarks of the lower esophageal sphincter are illustrated in Figure 1-3.

Studies focusing on pressure measurements and manometric determinations have provided useful information in the diagnosis and evaluation of motility disorders of the esophagus and the stomach. However, it has also become clear that pressure measurements do not predict clinically significant GE reflux.

## ASSESSMENT OF GER

The barium swallow and the upper GI series still represent the recommended initial study in the evaluation of recurrent vomiting. Anatomical anomalies such as malrotation, duodenal or antral webs, or a large hiatal hernia ("partial thoracic stomach") can be easily diagnosed. Serious pitfalls in management can then be avoided.

Because of the dissatisfaction encountered in the assessment of GE reflux with contrast x-rays and more sophisticated manometric studies using multiple-lumen transducers, a more meaningful test was sought involving prolonged esophageal pH monitoring. Glass or cadmium electrodes, at the tip of a size 3 French probe, can be left in position with a minimum of discomfort, even in the youngest patient. Avoiding the need for sedation is important since confounding artifacts could affect the measurements. Recordings can be carried out in the general pediatric floor, provided someone is available to record clinical events.

The accurate description of clinical occurrences during the course of the test has provided useful information when trying to answer questions about a suspected relation between GE reflux and apnea, wheezing, choking, cough, or pain from esophagitis (Fig 1–4).

The recording also provides information on the time needed to neutralize refluxed acid, a measure of the esophageal ''clearing mechanisms'' (peristalsis, saliva), which are considered important protective factors against acid and peptic injury.

Interpretation of the results is not always easy. A number of criteria have been proposed by various groups, bringing into account such features as duration of the *longest episode* with a pH below 4, the *number* of episodes with a pH below 4, *the percentage* of time spent at a pH below 4, and the mean duration of esophageal clearing. In addition, the course of reflux 2 hours following

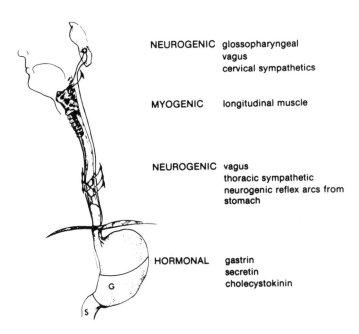

**FIG 1–2.**
The most important elements regulating swallowing and esophageal motility. (From Henderson RD: *The Esophagus: Reflux and Primary Disorders.* Baltimore, Williams & Wilkins Co, 1980. Used by permission.)

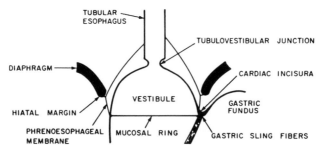

**FIG 1–3.**
Anatomical features of the lower esophageal sphincter. (From Castell DO, Wu WC, Ott DJ (eds): *Gastroesophageal Reflux Disease: Pathogenesis, Diagnosis, Therapy.* Mount Kisco, New York, Futura Publishing Co, 1985. Used by permission.)

ingestion of apple juice (acid) or milk (alkali) has been found helpful in distinguishing those children with gastroesophageal reflux disease.

Despite all the limitations and difficulties associated with the quantification of GE reflux by this method, prolonged observations offer a more realistic picture than a single view in time such as is given by an esophagogram or during a manometric study. Of all currently available methods of assessing GE reflux, pH monitoring remains the most informative, sensitive, and specific.

Recent advances in microelectronics permit the recording of the whole study on a small, portable tape which can then be displayed and analyzed by a computer program. The patient is free to engage in daily activities, and events such as pain, vomiting, etc., can be marked to be later displayed sequentially in graph form. The next few years will see an increase in the use of this technology because of the clear advantages it offers in avoiding hospitalization and because of the simplicity and good tolerance of the procedure.

## SCINTIGRAPHY

In recent years, the use of isotopes in the evaluation of gastroesophageal disorders has proliferated. Technetium 99m sulfur colloid can be added to milk or even solids such as eggs or meats, and a more physiological assessment of gastric emptying is possible.

Computerized analysis permits calculation of esophageal clearance and gastric emptying and detection of differences between solid and liquid phase emptying.

Aspiration of formula into the lungs can be documented if enough isotope remains in the stomach prior to the occurrence of reflux "over the top."

The dosage of radiation is small, and the method has found its supporters and enthusiasts. It can sometimes provide useful information, especially in the patient with impaired gastric motility where pyloroplasty is a serious consideration at the time of antireflux surgery.

## NATURAL HISTORY

It is important to understand the natural history of GE reflux. In over 70% of infants with GE reflux, the problem improves or resolves spontaneously by 18 months of age. During the first 3 months of life, the proportion of children with spontaneous symptomatic improvement is around 40%, so that in most cases the best approach is careful assessment and the use of temporizing measures as

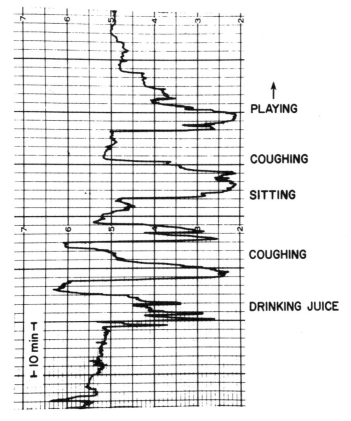

**FIG 1–4.**
Representative tracing of an intraesophageal pH monitoring. Note the association of coughing with several reflux episodes and the lack of symptoms during the last one despite similar changes. Esophageal clearance on this last episode is slightly prolonged.

described below. Esophageal strictures and death directly related to GE reflux has occurred in less than 5% in most series. In selected populations, such as found in institutions for the mentally retarded, GE reflux can be prevalent and tends to respond poorly to medical management.

## Management Pointers

There is a certain logic in attempting to improve reflux by thickening the feedings and maintaining the upright position, but in fact there are no studies that show conclusively that this is effective. Future systematic use of pH monitoring will allow more careful evaluation of the effect of accepted practices on the course of GE reflux. For example, for many years it was recommended to place the child in the sitting position in an adjustable "infant seat." Recent studies using continuous pH monitoring have shown that reflux episodes are more frequent and last longer when there is abdominal compression as occurs when the baby slouches. In the supine position, the GE junction in children tends to be anterior to the gastric bubble, thus favoring reflux.

On the other hand, radiologic studies have demonstrated that in the prone position, when the bed is in a 60-degree incline, the relative location of the GE junction and the fundic air bubble is optimal for minimizing reflux. As anyone who has tried to keep an infant in a tilted bed knows, it is often difficult if not impossible to prevent an older child from rolling and actually ending up head down. A parachute harness with Velcro attachments is at times useful in avoiding such rollover and is worth trying in the baby with troublesome reflux.*

Additional suggestions to the parents include:

1. Avoid giving liquids after the thickened feedings. This at times creates a "syphon" effect and favors reflux. (This is actually one of the techniques used by radiologists to elicit reflux!)

2. Limit the volume of the feedings to 4–6 ounces, rather than offering a full bottle at once. The rest of the bottle can be given an hour later, if needed for nutritional reasons.

3. Avoid juices since they are in most cases acidic (most apple juices have a pH of 4.5 or less), and can actually exacerbate esophagitis.

## ANTACIDS AND DRUGS AFFECTING MOTILITY

When more intensive intervention is necessary, there are several options that fall under the broad category of "medical management." Medications are used in an attempt to improve the function of the LES and to improve gastric emptying or decrease the irritating effects of acid contents on the esophageal mucosa. The most commonly used agents are the following.

* One version of the harness is available through MRI Corporation, Powell, Tennessee.

## Antacids

Gaviscon is an emulsion of aluminum hydroxide, magnesium carbonate, and sodium alginate and Xanthan gum. This preparation in its liquid form is more viscous and foamy, offering somewhat better surface adhesiveness and protection of the mucosa to the injurious effects of acid. Usually one teaspoon four times a day given 1–2 hours after feeding will offer relief if esophagitis is present.

Other antacids and simethicone-containing preparations will provide comparable benefits. Attention should be paid to common side effects seen with antacids, mainly loose stools or constipation.

## Improved LES Function

Bethanechol (Urocholine), commonly employed by urologists to increase the muscle tone of the urinary bladder, has been shown to increase the tone of the LES and to improve esophageal clearing. The daily dose recommended by Euler is 8.7 $mg/m^2$ in three or four divided doses. Side effects include nervousness, bladder spasm, diarrhea, tachycardia, and pallor.

Metoclopramide (Reglan), recently approved for use in the management of diabetic gastric stasis in adults and as an antiemetic in chemotherapy, offers several advantages over bethanechol. This dopamine antagonist, chemically related to the phenothiazines, not only increases the resting tone of the LES, but also relaxes the pylorus and the duodenum, increasing the synchronizing antral contractions. The end result is faster gastric emptying. The most worrisome side effect is the rare occurrence of extrapyramidal reactions (less than 1%), thought to occur more commonly in children than in adults. Patients with epilepsy are reported to be at even higher risk. Mitigating against this risk is the fact that the dosage used in children for control of GE reflux is 10–50 times smaller than the ones used in the control of nausea and vomiting during *cis*-platinum therapy. Diphenhydramine (Benadryl) is the antidote of choice when extrapyramidal reactions appear. Such reactions tend to subside after the medication is discontinued. More common side effects include irritability, somnolence, and diarrhea.

In infants with severe reflux, in whom x-ray studies have ruled out an anatomical problem (obstruction, large hiatal hernia), a cautious trial of metoclopramide (0.1 mg/kg dose 3 or 4 times a day) is justified if the child's health is being compromised by excessive loss of calories or severe esophagitis. Parents need to be informed of the potential side effects. Clinical studies are in progress, and this drug may soon be approved for the management of GE reflux in children. Newer "prokinetic" medications continue to be developed and investigated intensively. More specific action on the myenteric plexus and lack of extraintestinal side effects make these pharmacologic agents most promising.

*Indications for Surgery*

If, after trying all of the above measures, the patient's symptoms do not improve, consideration should be given to surgery. The major indications remain:

1. Failure to thrive.
2. Severe esophagitis or esophageal stricture.
3. Recurrent aspiration pneumonia, hyperreactive airway disease, or choking.
4. Barrett's esophagus (columnar-lined lower esophagus); premalignant in adults.
5. Sandifer's syndrome.

The Sandifer syndrome is a rare and peculiar condition characterized by bizarre neck and head movements, at times suggesting a primary neurological disorder such as dystonia. In some but not all patients, neck movements seem related to an involuntary attempt to minimize GE reflux. Response to antireflux surgery has been generally beneficial, although in some patients the head and neck movements have become an ingrained habit very difficult to eliminate.

The most common antireflux operation performed in the pediatric age group is the Nissen fundoplication. In this operation, the cardia is wrapped almost 360 degrees by the gastric fundus. This improves sphincter function by allowing gastric and intra-abdominal pressures to be transmitted circumferentially around the gastroesophageal sphincter (Fig 1–5).

In most procedures, the diaphragmatic crura are approximated to prevent slippage into the chest by excessive tension. Also, in most cases, a gastrostomy (temporary or permanent) will be included in the procedure. Recovery from surgery usually takes 5 to 7 days. Results of the Nissen fundoplication are usually very good, although not many long-term follow-up series have been reported.

The most commonly encountered complications of antireflux surgery include:

- Too tight a wrap with functional obstruction at the lower esophagus
- "Gas bloat" syndrome and inability to vomit
- Injury to the vagus nerve with disordered motility and pyloric dysfunction
- Dumping syndrome, which may be troublesome and difficult to manage
- Slipped Nissen with recurrence (inadvertent) of reflux and its dangers.

## BIBLIOGRAPHY

1. Castell DO, Wu WC, Ott DJ (eds): *Gastroesophageal Reflux Disease*. Mount Kisko, New York, Futura Publishing Co, 1985.
2. Henderson RD: *The Esophagus: Reflux and Primary Motor Disorders*. Baltimore, Williams & Wilkins Co, 1980.
3. Herbst JJ: Gastroesophageal reflux. *J Pediatr* 1981; 98 (6):859–870.

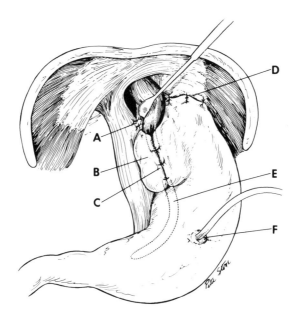

**FIG 1–5.**
Salient features of Nissen fundoplication in infants. **A**, crural sutures to reduce hiatus. **B**, generous loose, adequate tissue in the wrap. **C**, sutures placed through seromuscular depth of both gastric and esophageal walls. **D**, sutures to fix the fundus to the diaphragm. **E**, appropriate sized mercury-filled dilator to ensure adequate lumen. **F**, gastrostomy in all infants and whenever there is any question of gastric outlet problems. (From Randolph JG: 1983; *Ann Surg* 198:579–584. Used by permission.)

4. Balistreri WF, Farrell MK: Gastroesophageal reflux in infants (editorial). *N Engl J Med* 1983; 309(13):790–792.
5. Euler AR: Use of bethanechol for the treatment of gastroesophageal reflux. *J Pediatr* 1980; 96:321–124.
6. Schulze KD: Metoclopramide. *N Engl J Med* 1981; 305(1):28–33.
7. Jamieson GG, Duranceau, AC: The defense mechanisms of the esophagus. *Surg Clin North Am* 1983; 63(4):787–799.
8. Piepsz A, Georges B, Rodesch, P, et al: Gastroesophageal scinti-scanning in children. *J Nucl Med* 1982; 23:631.
9. Orenstein SR, Lofton SW, Orenstein DM: Bethanechol for pediatric gastroesophageal reflux: A prospective, blind, controlled study. *J Pediatr Gastroenterol Nutr* 1986; 5:549–555.
10. Arasu TS, Wyllie R, Fitzgerald JF, et al: Gastroesophageal reflux in infants and children: Comparative accuracy of diagnostic methods. *J Pediatr* 1980; 96(5)798–803.

# 2

# Failure to Thrive

The identification of normal growth is probably one of the most reassuring experiences for both parents and physicians. Recognition of an infant's progression along expected percentile curves, for weight and height as well as for head circumference, is an important sign of good health. Developmental milestones, psychomotor maturation, and socialization complement the general picture of the growing child and provide a frame of reference to measure the severity of many commonly encountered childhood problems: feeding difficulties, diarrhea, vomiting, infections.

No two children will grow in the exact same way. Genetic endowment, nutritional diversity, environmental demands, and social factors will have their share of influence in the final result. In many instances, the child shows an amazing resilience in the face of adversity and is able to overcome periods of disturbed growth with accelerated and more effective tissue synthesis, if only a window of opportunity is open.

## MONITORING GROWTH

As varied as growth and development are, it is still possible to have reasonable expectations and to monitor a child's progress with the help of very simple tools. The growth curve remains one of the most important instruments in the practitioner's armamentarium. Understanding the information contained in those percentile curves allows early detection of abnormal patterns and can offer reassurance in the face of what parents consider inadequate height or weight gains.

Some of the most commonly used curves are the ones developed by the National Center for Health Statistics (NCHS Standards). These curves represent contemporary (1979) norms for American children of same age and sex. Corrections for particular geographic, racial, and economic population subsets are possible from available NCHS documents.

Two standard deviations from the 50th percentile are represented by the 3rd percentile curve and, by definition, children in that lower curve are still "within normal limits." Not infrequently a child will fall slightly off the weight percentile curve at around age 9–12 months, and then resume growth along a new track.

Birth weight and the weight in the first few months of life are more a reflection of the intrauterine environment than true expression of one's genetically determined program. Once a child has been growing in a given percentile curve, a change to a *higher* curve is also abnormal. If the change is only in weight percentile, exogenous obesity is the most common reason. Of greater concern, however, is an acceleration in linear growth, since this might represent excess growth hormone from a pituitary adenoma or other endocrine abnormalities.

## FAILURE TO THRIVE

The term "failure to thrive" is used to describe the abnormal (or supposedly abnormal) pattern of growth in children less than 3 years old. Other terms, such as delayed growth, growth failure, and delayed sexual maturation are more commonly applied to older children and teenagers. What is being described is the discrepancy between the observed and the expected rates of weight and height gains.

It is obvious, and often taken for granted, that accurate and consistent measurements are crucial if the detection of abnormal velocities is going to be reliable. Extrapolation of measurements made at short intervals (i.e., less than 1 year) is inaccurate, since the tables are based on yearly observations. Weight measurements are usually more reproducible than heights. A good scale is sound investment for the pediatrician and practitioner. It is more difficult to obtain an accurate length in a moving infant. The degree of leg extension (which should not be forced), the position of the head on the examining table, and the flatness of the whole body on the table can easily add or subtract 2 to 3 cm. To minimize these artifacts, it is useful to place the child on a measuring board, another worthwhile investment if one considers the consequences of the misdiagnosis of failure to thrive. Standing height is usually about 2.0 cm less than supine length in infants and 1 cm less after age 4 years, and is easy to measure with a stadiometer.

*Diagnosis*

Assuming accurate measurements, a diagnosis of failure to thrive should not be made until the trend has been confirmed by at least three time points over a period of 2 to 3 months. Depending on the clinical picture, what is initially referred to as failure to thrive is often acute malnutrition. The practitioner should be able to suspect one or the other on the basis of the pattern of abnormalities.

A useful concept in the assessment of growth is the *weight for height ratio or percent*. By extrapolating the observed height to the 50th percentile curve, the *height age* is determined. The *weight age or standard weight* is then defined as the expected weight for a child whose height is at the 50th percentile. The ratio of the actual child's weight and the standard weight $\times$ 100 gives a measure of the proportional loss of body mass compared to height. For example, (Fig 2–1) if a 15-month-old infant girl presented with a weight of 6.5 kg and a length of 70 cm, her height age would be 9 months, at which age she should weigh 8.6 kg. The % wt/ht is 6.5/8.6 $\times$ 100, or 75% (Fig 2–2). Values below 80% are strongly suggestive of serious protein-calorie malnutrition. On the back of the NCHS charts, there is a percentile distribution plotting of the weights for heights of infants and prepubescent boys and girls. Values below the 5th percentile are interpreted in a similar way.

*Clinical Patterns*

By considering the weight, the height (or length), and the head circumference, three major patterns can be appreciated:

1. small head circumference, decreased weight, *and* height.
2. normal head circumference, disproportionate height, and weight close to normal.
3. normal head circumference, normal height, and decreased weight.

The first pattern reflects a basic abnormality of growth and is most suggestive of an intrauterine insult or a genetic (chromosomal) defect. Many of these children are small for dates, or small for gestational age (SGA), suggesting that inhibitory influences started acting prior to delivery. Since poor growth of the head reflects poor growth of the brain, many of these children also suffer from neurological deficits secondary to certain inborn errors of metabolism (producing hypoglycemia, for example) or fetal infection with viruses or toxoplasma.

The retardation of somatic growth must be explained in the broader context, since attempts at weight gain might result in further aberrations. Many of these children will become extremely obese if caloric requirements are not adjusted for the degree of activity and linear growth. Since in many instances the physician will be called to advise about ways to improve the growth of these children, a sense of proportion is necessary to offer realistic expectations and adequate nutritional guidelines.

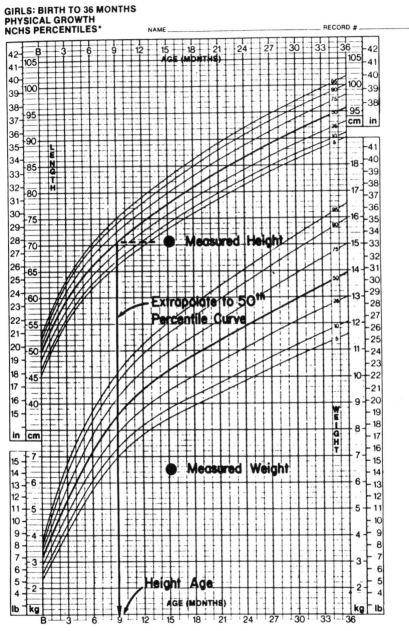

**GIRLS: BIRTH TO 36 MONTHS**
**PHYSICAL GROWTH**
**NCHS PERCENTILES***

NAME _____  RECORD # _____

**FIG 2–1.**
Having plotted the measured weight and height, the height is extrapolated to the 50th percentile curve to determine the weight-age. (From Hamill PVV, et al: Physical growth: National Center for Health Statistics Percentiles. *Am J Clin Nutr* 1979; 32:607–629. Courtesy of Ross Laboratories, Columbus, Ohio.)

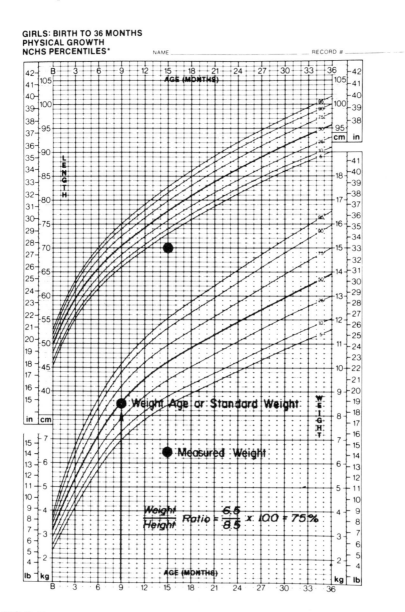

**FIG 2–2.**
The weight-age or standard weight is the appropriate 50th percentile weight for the height-age. The ratio is then calculated between the standard weight and the measured weight. See text. (From Hamill PVV, et al: Physical growth: National Center for Health Statistics Percentiles. *Am J Clin Nutr* 1979; 32:607–629. Courtesy of Ross Laboratories, Columbus, Ohio.)

On the other hand, when linear growth is preferentially affected, the major considerations are endocrinopathies and bone or cartilage growth abnormalities. Various dwarfism syndromes will present with this combination of normal head circumference, normal weight age, and disproportionate legs and/or arms.

Measurement of the upper (US) and lower (LS) segments, from the head to the symphysis pubis, and from there to the feet, respectively, is useful for detecting these patterns of growth abnormalities. The US–LS ratio in the infant is 1.7–1.8:1 and becomes closer to 1.0–0.9:1 as the child matures and reaches ages 10 and 18 years, respectively. Persistence of US–LS ratios in the infantile range strongly suggest interference with linear growth. This can be seen in hypothyroidism, hypopituitarism, or achondroplasia. Advanced US–LS ratio can be found in progeria or in precocious puberty syndromes.

Finally, a disproportionately low weight for height with normal head circumference immediately suggests malnutrition and requires a more complete investigation, as will be outlined subsequently. In the face of chronic hypocaloric intake, head and linear growth are preferentially preserved. If starvation is long lasting, both measurements will eventually suffer.

The consequences of prolonged malnutrition in the developing infant have always been a major concern of modern pediatrics, and a subtle loss of intellectual and social abilities has been detected in follow-up studies. Animal experiments have shown a wide range of brain cell abnormalities and a decrease in total brain DNA and protein when severe restriction of calories and protein occurs during the crucial period of brain growth. In humans, this period is in the first 2 years of life; hence, the importance of prompt recognition and investigation of any infant with failure to gain weight adequately.

## A STEPWISE APPROACH TO THE CHILD WITH MALNUTRITION

It has been said and proven time and time again that the most important aspect of the workup of the child with failure to thrive is the clinical history.

Based on the facts elicited during a thorough and systematic history complemented by a detailed physical examination, the range of possibilities can be narrowed to a few pertinent ones, and confirmatory tests then specifically ordered. In many cases, following the initial assessment, a diagnostic (and often therapeutic) trial can be instituted, sometimes as an outpatient, depending on the degree of malnutrition or on the suspicions and concerns of the physician.

Indiscriminate ordering of tests is to be discouraged, since the yield is nil when the clinical history does not suggest the diagnosis in the first place. In a retrospective study, in only 1.4% of 2,500 tests ordered in the workup of 185 children hospitalized with failure to thrive was the test helpful in offering a specific diagnosis; in each case, the study was indicated on clinical grounds.

## THE FOUR BASIC QUESTIONS

The four basic questions in the evaluation of the child with malnutrition are:
1. Is the intake adequate (quantity and quality)?
2. Is absorption and digestion normal?
3. Are requirements unusually high?
4. Is the parent-child interaction nurturing?

## INADEQUATE CALORIC INTAKE

A dietary history starts with a recall of all foodstuffs consumed in a representative 3- to 7-day period. For the infant, this is easier than in the older child, where estimate of the portions of solids is less accurate. Even more difficult is the assessment of nutritional intake in the breast-fed infant who fails to thrive. Weighing before and after a feed is not an ideal way of evaluating intake in this situation, but can offer a rough estimate. At times, it might become necessary to express the milk to have a better idea of the amounts produced. Again, this is less efficient than a sucking infant and can be deceiving. In other instances, analysis of the breast milk for electrolytes might be important in view of the occasional occurrence of hyponatremia and hypochloremic alkalosis (chloride deficiency syndrome) which results in anorexia and impaired growth.

It is important to inquire about the specifics of formula preparation. Inadvertent errors in dilution can result in a hypodense formula or diarrhea and malabsorption if a concentrate is given straight from the can. Reasons for such errors should be explored. At times, they reflect serious financial difficulties in the household, while in other cases it might result from the desire to promote better than normal growth, without realizing the consequences of offering undiluted formula.

If the amount of formula and solids is theoretically sufficient to promote normal weight gain, the next question concerns whether the food is actually being consumed and retained. Feeding difficulties and excessive vomiting can seriously curtail the total caloric intake. In fact, *poor intake is probably the most frequent reason for malnutrition in infants.* Is this in turn a result of central nervous system dysfunction? Is there choking and coughing in association with the feedings? Is a tracheoesophageal fistula present? Nasal regurgitation of formula suggests dyscoordinated swallowing, cleft palate, or massive GE reflux.

Does the child drink eagerly, only to vomit immediately or hours later? Pyloric spasm and hypertrophic pyloric stenosis can present with semiacute malnutrition and dehydration.

Other important anatomical abnormalities to be considered in the differential diagnosis of significant vomiting are the intestinal stenoses, malrotation, volvulus, and aganglionosis.

Extraintestinal etiologies of vomiting which need to be sought for and ruled out on clinical and laboratory grounds include CNS tumors (with or without increased intracranial pressure) and renal defects resulting in metabolic derangements or mechanical obstruction (ureteropelvic or ureterocystic occlusion, stones, glomerulonephritis, polycystic kidneys). Inborn errors of carbohydrate and protein metabolism can present with anorexia and vomiting, and a high index of suspicion is needed to correlate the dietary history with the onset and evolution of the symptoms.

Anorexia is often a prominent feature of the clinical picture of failure to thrive. Refusal to eat can be simply a psychological response to a tense and upsetting feeding experience or can be a sign of more serious pathology. Any chronic illness, whether renal, pulmonary, cardiac or neurologic can result in decreased interest in food. The presence of a malignancy has sometimes dramatic effects on caloric intake, well before the problem is compounded by the side effects of medications and radiotherapy. Malnutrition per se, such as results from chronic diarrhea and malabsorption of any origin, will often be accompanied by anorexia. Ketosis from starvation will produce nausea and prolong nutritional rehabilitation.

## ABNORMAL DIGESTION AND ABSORPTION

The subject is covered in detail in Chapter 4.

Important clues of impaired digestion and malabsorption include:

1. Diarrhea
2. Steatorrhea
3. Foul-smelling stools
4. Bloatedness
5. Vomiting
6. Skin manifestation of vitamin and micronutrient deficiency
   a. Cheilosis
   b. Glossitis
   c. Dermatitis
   d. Nail and hair dysplasia
   e. Bruising
   f. Photophobia

7. Muscle wasting and weakness
8. Hepatomegaly secondary to steatosis (fatty liver).

## ABNORMAL REQUIREMENTS

Determining energy expenditure and abnormal intermediate metabolism is still a difficult question to answer in practical terms. Devices able to accurately measure oxygen consumption are in use in research institutions, and much information is being gathered on the metabolic demands of the low birth weight infants. The instrumentation needed does not lend itself to immediate application to the older child, so that in most cases, the assessment of increased metabolic requirements is an estimate rather than a verified fact.

The *energy cost of growth* is the number of calories needed to deposit a gram of tissue. The value that has been estimated based on balance studies in infants less than 3 months of age is around 4.5 gm to 7.5 gm for 100 kcal. This can only be used as rough guide to gauge the adequacy of weight gain when caloric intake is known with certainty. In other words, a healthy 5-kg infant receiving 600 kcal/day should reasonably be expected to gain about 30 gm/day. Many factors affect this estimate, including the degree of activity, age, and state of nutrition. Taking the weight gain curve at the 50th percentile, an expected rate of gain for the first 6 months of life calculates at approximately 3.5 gm/100 kcal, while it is half this figure for the rest of the first year.

When a child does not gain weight at these expected rates, the two major issues revolve around the questions (1) are abnormal metabolic requirements present? or (2) are strong psychosocial inhibitions responsible for the failure to thrive?

The most common reasons for increased metabolic demands include:

• Excessive activity
• Fever
• Infection
• Trauma, including surgery
• Chronic renal failure
• Chronic heart disease
• Pulmonary insufficiency
• Cirrhosis
• Malignancy
• Endocrine abnormalities (hyperthyroidism, diabetes, hypercorticism)
• Excessive losses (malabsorption syndromes, nephrotic syndrome)
• Abnormal intermediate metabolism (inborn errors of amino acid, carbohydrate, and organic acid metabolism)

- Central nervous system disease (dystonias and other movement disorders, diencephalic syndrome, myopathies).

## DISTURBED PARENT-CHILD INTERACTION

In the evaluation of the child with poor weight gain, one of the most important considerations, once the physician has thoroughly performed a review of systems and concluded after the physical examination that no obvious physical problem exists, is to determine the psychodynamics of the parent-child relationship. Remembering that the common denominator in most nonorganic failure to thrive is a lack of adequate intake, the factors responsible for this end result should be sought. A great deal of patience and compassion is needed to elicit sensitive material. More than one interview is often necessary to build a rapport of trust with the family.

Issues that contribute to abnormalities in the attachment of a parent to their infant include:

- Age
- Emotional maturity of the parents
- Circumstances of the pregnancy (unwanted, illicit, adulterous, incestuous)
- Depression
- Alcoholism and other drug abuse
- Matrimonial disharmony
- Mental illness (phobias and other neuroses, psychoses)
- Family stress (financial, social).

It is important not to project an accusatory attitude by implying that the problem with the child's poor growth is due to the parent's shortcomings or inadequacies. Unless obvious neglect or abuse are apparent, the physician should withhold judgment until he or she has had a first-hand opportunity to witness the family situation and the parents' background.

Frequently a child with a serious feeding difficulty will thoroughly depress even the best-prepared and loving parent. Inexperience, pressure from family and friends, and other circumstances beyond the parents' control can result in disturbed relationships and a tense household. Loneliness, a sense of frustration, insecurity, and tiredness from sleepless nights can combine to create a very distorted image of the parent and should not make the practitioner jump to conclusions. In many instances, more is gained by guidance and open discussion on what the normal processes of child growth and development are than by putting the parents on the defensive and contributing to their poor self-esteem.

## Management

Following the stepwise approach described in the preceding pages, a systematic evaluation of the components determining the growth equation (intake, metabolism, losses, psyche) will give a general overview of the possible etiologies of the failure to thrive. Again, use of the growth chart and judicious interpretation of the measurements is crucial and will save a great deal in unnecessary anxiety and concern.

If a specific diagnosis is suggested, confirmatory laboratory work is completed and treatment instituted, be it a change in diet (lactose-free, cow's protein-free, low fat, etc.), a nutritional supplement (bicarbonate, iron, zinc, etc.), or medication (digitalis, metoclopramide, or steroid replacement).

### *In-Hospital Evaluation*

When decreased intake is suspected, and the circumstances are not entirely clear from the history, a diagnostic and therapeutic trial should be carried out in the hospital.

A minimum of laboratory tests are usually necessary at this stage, and should mainly screen for metabolic disorders and other indices of prolonged nutrient deficiency (for example, anemia or hypoalbuminemia). Serum electrolytes and complete blood count are useful in the child with recurrent infections and diarrhea, as some children with neutropenia will present with failure to thrive. Anemia and microcytosis can also be easily detected. The demonstration of a concentrated urine in the morning, or a urine with pH of 5 helps rule out some of the tubular disorder resulting in chronic acidosis. A sweat test is indicated in any child with chronic diarrhea and failure to thrive, even if pulmonary symptoms are absent. The presence of anemia, edema, and FTT should heighten the possibility of CF. Many of these infants are breast-fed, and diarrhea can be prominent or subtle. The investigation of vomiting and GE reflux has been covered in Chapter 1.

Observation by the nursing staff of the whole feeding process and documentation of the volume consumed, the time and difficulties encountered, and the child's response should be done reliably. Identification of the areas of difficulty (sucking, swallowing, excessive regurgitation, irritability, abnormal posturing, etc.) should be followed by attempts to correct the problems by teaching proper techniques and compensating for the losses or limiting the intake.

## BIBLIOGRAPHY

1. Sills RH: Failure to thrive: The role of clinical and laboratory evaluation. *Am J Dis Child* 1978; 132:967–969.
2. Hannaway PJ: Failure to thrive: A study of 100 infants. *Clin Pediatr* 1970; 9:96–99.

3. Hamill PVV, et al: Physical growth: National Center for Health Statistics Percentiles. *Am J Clin Nutr* 1979; 32:607–629.
4. Hufton IW, Ates KR: Non-organic failure to thrive: A long term follow-up. *Pediatrics* 1977; 59:73–77.
5. Chase HP, Martin HPV: Undernutrition and child development. *N Engl J Med* 1970; 282:933.
6. Goldbloom RB: Failure to thrive. *Pediatr Clin North Am* 1982; 29:151.
7. Suskind RM, Varma RN: Assessment of nutritional status of children. *Pediatr Rev* 1983; 5:195.
8. Pollitt E, Eichler A: Behavioral disturbances among failure to thrive children. *Am J Dis Child* 1976; 130:24–28.
9. Cupoli JM, Hallock JA, Barness LA: Failure to thrive. *Curr Probl Pediatr* 1980; 10(11):1–43.
10. Rosenn D, Loeb L, Jura M: Differentiation of organic from nonorganic failure to thrive syndrome in infancy. *Pediatrics* 1980; 66:689.
11. Woolston JL: Eating disorders in infancy and early childhood. *J Am Acad Child Psychiatr* 1983; 22:114.
12. Chatoor I, Egan J: Nonorganic failure to thrive and dwarfism due to food refusal: A separation disorder. *J Am Acad Child Psychiatr* 1983; 22:294.
13. Smith DW, Truog W, Rogers JE, et al: Shifting linear growth during infancy: Illustration of genetic factors in growth from fetal life through infancy. *J Pediatr* 1976; 89:225.

# 3

# Investigation of Gastrointestinal Disorders

The management of the patient with gastrointestinal disease can be enhanced by the routine application of a few basic and easy-to-perform tests. The methods can be learned (and taught) in a few minutes, and the instrumentation needed is available in most offices already: slides, tubes, droppers, microscope. The reagents also are easy to obtain, and the information provided after a few minutes of work is more than worth the time required to perform the tests.

Office investigation of malabsorption or suspected liver disease is, on the other hand, more involved and often requires special equipment and trained personnel. In most cases, those patients will be referred to a specialist who can coordinate the workup.

Centralized laboratories have evolved in the past decade that are able to provide fast and usually reliable service to a large base of practitioners. The range of routine tests that can now be ordered and the development of microtechniques have allowed broad biochemical screening from very small blood samples. Information gathered incidentally during "routine" testing is responsible for a great deal of surprises, concerns, and repeat tests. Nonetheless, available services to the practitioner offer a practical and convenient mechanism to initiate the investigation of the patient suspected of having a gastrointestinal problem, whether inflammatory bowel disease or failure to thrive. Familiarity with the tests available, with the normal ranges for age, physiological meaning, and sensitivity, is crucial for accurate interpretation.

## IMMEDIATELY AVAILABLE METHODS FOR STOOL TESTING

### Using All Senses

The firmness or looseness of the stool, its color, and smell are always of great interest to parents and is a frequent source of concern and bewilderment. Expectations and descriptions vary so much that direct inspection by the physician can be the only way to obtain a more objective description.

Witnessing a bowel movement in an infant can be most informative, not only for assessing the difficulties associated with its passage but also for documenting explosive expulsion or frothing, both suggestive of fermentation of malabsorbed substrate (mainly carbohydrate or fat). The bulkiness seen during consumption of high fiber diets should not be confused with steatorrhea, which is also accompanied by a foul smell representing bacterial decomposition of proteins, starches, and fat. The rancid, putrid smell of a malabsorptive stool is not easily forgotten. Parents should be questioned whether the smell is so offensive as to require ventilating the bathroom or the whole house!

The stool should also be inspected for the presence of blood. Fresh streaking on the surface suggests a fissure or polyp. Blood mixed within mucoid stools is more commonly seen in colitis or proctitis. To confirm the presence of blood is simple with one of the guaiac impregnated cards, developed with a peroxide solution right in the office (see under ''GI bleeding''). Melanotic stools of upper GI bleeds, maroon stools of a Meckel's diverticulum, or bright red blood of a colonic lesion should be inspected first hand since they have such serious implications. The ''currant jelly'' stools of prolonged intussusception represents intestinal mucus mixed with venous blood resulting from vascular compromise and edema. The purulent stools of dysentery and other inflammatory diseases of the rectum and colon are also characteristic, and their recognition is of diagnostic importance.

### Microscopic Examination of the Stool

With a cotton swab, stool is rolled gently on glass slides and allowed to air dry. Sampling should be from the mucus-containing portions rather than from the solid part. Once dried, it is very easy to stain the slides with a solution of Metylene Blue for microscopic inspection. With this stain, or with a conventional Wright-Giemsa such as is commonly used in hematology, polymorphonuclears are easily identified. Sheets of polys are seen in enteropathogenic bacterial gastroenteritis and in inflammatory colitis (Fig 3–1). The Wright-Giemsa stain is necessary for recognition of eosinophils and Charcot-Leyden crystals. The latter are thought to represent fragments of destroyed eosinophils. Their presence suggests protein allergy, although it can also be seen in inflammations of the colon.

## Identification of Fat and Starch

Qualitative determination of fat in the stool is not a reliable method of investigating suspected steatorrhea. The usefulness of the test is more in helping confirm the presence of fat in a stool that appears suspicious, either because of its light color, bulkiness, or oiliness. It is also of some help in following the response to refeeding after prolonged diarrhea or in the patient with cholestasis.

A small dab of stool is mixed with a couple of drops of saline on a slide. One or two drops of sudan red stain is then stirred in, and the specimen is covered with a glass slide. Fat droplets appear pink in color and can be single or conglomerated, large or small in size (see Fig 3–1).

To detect starch, the same procedure is used with iodine solution as the stain. It is normal to see undigested fiber in the stool, and this test has very little application today. Larger amounts of starch (intra- and extracellular) can be seen in pancreatic insufficiency (see Fig 3–1).

It is more difficult to develop the confidence to identify the most common parasites, *Giardia lamblia* and *Entamoeba histolytica*. Everyone remembers the familiar pictures of *Giardia* looking like a mustachioed cell with two pairs of eyes (see Fig 4–5, p 45), but few practitioners would actually recognize it if they saw it eye to eye. A little practice is all it takes. If a microscope is available in the office, a more reliable examination can be carried out, since a fresh specimen is usually available after the rectal examination. It is possible to fix the stool in polyvinyl alcohol, so that lysis of the organisms does not take place during transport. If so collected, the stool can remain refrigerated (not frozen) for 1 to 3 days without affecting the yield. Trichrome and iron hematoxylin are good stains for identification of *Giardia*. Special flotation techniques can be used for better separation of the cysts and trophozoites, but this is not very practical in the usual office setting and the physician should depend on a reliable parasitology laboratory when these diagnoses are considered.

## Identifying Carbohydrate Malabsorption

The presence of sugar in the stool often reflects damage to the intestinal villi after a bout of gastroenteritis. More rarely, it can result from congenital deficiencies of the disaccharidases responsible for hydrolysis of carbohydrate. Iden-

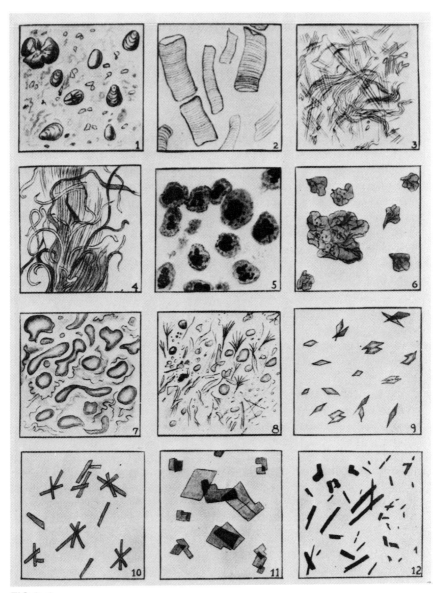

**FIG 3–1.**
Some of the most common findings in the microscopic examination of stool. Special stains (i.e., iodine for starch, Wright-Giemsa or methylene blue for fecal leukocytes) greatly help in identification. **1**, undigested starch granules. **2**, partly digested muscle. **3**, connective tissue. **4**, elastic tissue. **5**, neutrophilic leukocytes. **6**, epithelial cells. **7**, neutral fat. **8**, fatty acid and soap crystals. **9**, Charcot-Leyden crystals. **10**, hematoidin crystals. **11**, cholesterin crystals. **12**, bismuth oxide crystals. (From Kolmer JA, Spaulding EH, Robinson HW: *Approved Laboratory Technic.* New York, Appleton-Century-Crofts, 1951. Used by permission.)

tifying sugars that have a reducing group (glucose, fructose, galactose, lactose, and maltose) is of great importance in the practical management of the child with diarrhea. Sucrose is not a reducing sugar, and a negative test for reducing substances while consuming this sugar is not meaningful unless the stool has been boiled with hydrochloric acid (1N) for at least 20 minutes.

The method for checking reducing substances in the stool is another application of the Benedict reaction between copper sulfate and the reducing sugar group in the presence of sodium citrate. Sodium hydroxide is present to generate heat. The presence of this strong base makes proper use and storage of the tablets important to avoid burns. The most commonly used method employs the Clinitest tablets (Ames, Elkhart, Indiana), originally developed for the detection of sugar in the urine. The tablets should be kept in a dark and dry place and should be used within their stated expiration date.

The method is semiquantitative, based on a color scale provided in the product insert. The range is expressed in + units, from 1 to 4, which roughly represent $1/4$ to 2 gm%. The test can be done in a plastic tube, such as the ones commonly used for urine analysis. The liquid part of the diarrheal stool should be used, remembering that the new disposable diapers are very effective in absorbing the stool water. If necessary, the diaper should be squeezed over the test tube. If the stool is formed, about 1 gm should be stirred with 10 drops of water. The tablet is added and the reaction allowed to proceed without further stirring or shaking. After 15 seconds, the color is read and compared to the chart.

When sugar is malabsorbed and reaches the colon, bacterial hydrolysis and metabolism generates organic acids, lowering the stool pH. Normal stool pH is around 7–8, depending on the diet. During breast feeding or in premature infants, stool tends to be more acidic, and it has been postulated that this favors colonization with enteroprotective lactobacilli. Low stool pH (3–5) is often seen in carbohydrate malabsorption. Determination is immediate with a pH strip, such as Nitrazine paper (Squibb and Sons, Princeton, New Jersey) which covers the range 4.5 (yellow)–7.5 (blue). Again, the pH should be measured on the liquid portion of the stool. If stool cannot be brought for testing within 1–2 hours, it should be frozen to prevent carbohydrate breakdown by bacteria and false negative test for reducing substances. In the hospital, stools can be preserved with an acid solution of 0.04% sodium fluoride. This inhibits glycolysis almost completely.

### Breath Hydrogen Testing

This technique takes advantage of the fact that bacteria generate hydrogen during the metabolism of carbohydrates and other substrates. There is no human biochemical reaction that produces hydrogen as a byproduct. A segment of the population (as high as 4%) does not have hydrogen-producing bacteria. In those individuals, the breath hydrogen test will not be useful, giving false negative results.

If the patient has hydrogen-producing bacteria in the gut, the breath hydrogen test is sensitive and reproducible. Although not quantitative, the test is useful and easily performed. It should always be correlated with clinical symptoms of intolerance and, if possible, stool testing for reducing substances and pH.

The test consists of collecting aliquots of expired air during a period of time, usually 2 to 3 hours. Older children can be taught to breathe in the collecting apparatus while infants can have the test done with soft nasal prongs or a nasal catheter. The instrument for hydrogen detection and quantitation (as parts per million) is now available in compact units whose thermal or liquid gas chromatograph is dedicated to hydrogen measurements and requires little maintenance. It is not likely that the practitioner will do carbohydrate tolerance testing in his or her office, but being aware of this methodology and realizing its potential is an important step in considering the possibility of documenting suspected intolerances. With this information in hand, the planning of an elimination diet involves less guesswork, and unnecessary restrictions are not imposed on the basis of assumption alone.

Other applications of breath testing involve determination of transit time using a nonabsorbable carbohydrate such as lactulose (an artificial galactose-fructose disaccharide) or detection of bacterial overgrowth. The presence of bacteria in the small intestine causes an early rise in hydrogen production, which can be detected in timed collections of expired air. Bacterial overgrowth can be responsible for malabsorption in conditions of deranged peristalsis, incompetent ileocecal valve (surgical removal, inflammatory bowel disease), or congenital abnormalities such as enteric duplications or acquired internal fistulae.

## Quantitative Fat Measurements

When steatorrhea is suspected, a timed collection of the stool (usually 3 days) will permit quantitation of unabsorbed fat. Knowing the fat intake makes determination of the *coefficient of absorption* a simple calculation. (Excreted fat (gm)/consumed fat (gm) × 100). In practice, charcoal or carmine red markers should be given at the beginning and end of the 72-hour collection period. A teaspoon or two of charcoal slurry is usually sufficient. Parents should be asked to keep a food diary, and instructed to give high-fat foodstuffs. A practical suggestion is to use a bar of butter or margarine during the period of the test. This ensures a more reliable fat intake. The stool is collected in a preweighed jar or paint can, and until completion of the collection the container should be kept refrigerated (and tightly sealed).

## Xylose Tolerance Test

D-xylose is a 5-carbon sugar absorbed by passive diffusion directly into the small intestine (duodenum and jejunum mainly), without participation of the lymphatics. Its absorption thus reflects the enterocyte area. The xylose tolerance test is useful for the screening and monitoring of patients with malabsorption secondary to villus atrophy. In the past, the test involved a 5-hour urine collection, but validation in children has shown the 1- and 2-hour serum levels are reliable indicators of absorptive function.

The xylose is administered as a 10% solution after an overnight fast. It should be consumed in a brief period of time. Ideally, intraduodenal or intragastric administration (if gastric emptying is normal) should minimize errors associated with erratic ingestion. Only a small amount of blood is needed for xylose determination, preferably obtained by venipuncture. Nomograms exist for plotting the values obtained at 1 and 2 hours. A serum level of 30 mg% or higher is reassuring, while values below 25 mg% suggest villus damage. This then needs to be confirmed by other methods, including jejunal biopsy.

## Jejunal Biopsy

This test remains in the realm of the specialist, but its usefulness should also be realized by the practitioner. The procedure usually requires hospitalization, although older patients can have it as outpatients, especially if heavy sedation is not used. In the younger child, premedication with a "lytic cocktail" such as the popular Demerol:Phenergan:Thorazine, 1 mg/kg each, will usually suffice. Use of a steerable catheter makes the procedure quick (just a few minutes) in contrast with the Crosby capsule, which has to pass into the jejunum by itself, propelled by peristalsis after negotiating the pylorus.

Sampling of duodenal contents for culture and pancreatic enzyme determination is also possible once the intubation is successful. The sample of tissue is sufficient for microscopic examination and for disaccharidase determination. The test is only done after normal coagulation and platelets have been documented. It is not a high-risk procedure, and complications such as perforation and bleeding are extremely rare.

The major indications for jejunal biopsy appear in Table 3–1.

## BIBLIOGRAPHY

1. Ahlquist DA, McGill DB, Schwartz, S, et al: Hemoquant, a new quantitative assay for fecal hemoglobin: Comparison with hemoccult. *Ann Intern Med* 1984; 101:297–302.
2. Vanderhoof JA, Hunt LI, Antonson DL: A rapid procedure for small intestinal biopsy in infants and children. *Gastroenterology* 1981; 80:938–941.

TABLE 3–1.

Indications for Jejunal Biopsy

---

For diagnosis of
    Gluten-induced enteropathy
    Abetalipoproteinemia
    Intestinal Lymphangiectasia
    Confirmation of Disaccharidase deficiency
        Lactase
        Sucrase — Isomaltase
To confirm villus abnormality in
    Protracted diarrhea
    Protein allergies
    Tropical sprue
    Immunoglobulin deficiency syndromes

---

3. Russell RI, Lee TD: Tests of small intestinal function: Digestion, absorption, secretion. *Clin Gastroenterol* 1978; 7:277–315.
4. Christie DL: Use of the one-hour blood xylose test as an indicator of small bowel mucosal disease. *J. Pediatr* 1978; 92:725–728.
5. Ghosh SK, Littlewood JM, Goddard D, et al: Stool microscopy in screening for steatorrhoea. *J Clin Pathol* 1977; 30:749.
6. Rubin CE, Dobbins WO, III: Peroral biopsy of the small intestine: A review of its diagnostic usefulness. *Gastroenterology* 1965; 49:676.
7. Barr RG, Perman JA, Schoeller DA, et al: Breath tests in pediatric gastrointestinal disorders: New diagnostic opportunities. *Pediatrics* 1978; 62(3):393–401.
8. King CE, Toskes PP: The use of breath tests in the study of malabsorption. *Clin Gastroenterol* 1983; 12:591–610.

# 4

# Malabsorption

The process of digestion and absorption of foodstuffs has been described in detail in recent reviews, and the reader should keep up to date with the constantly evolving picture of the physiological mechanisms involved. A good understanding of all factors will improve the diagnostic skills by providing a firm basis for interpreting abnormal findings and tailoring the workup.

In brief, the major elements contributing to normal digestion and absorption of nutrients are:

1. Intact gastrointestinal tract (anatomically and functionally).
2. Normal brush border enzymes.
3. Normal emulsification, translocation, and processing of dietary fats.
4. Normal pancreatic function.

It is not difficult to end up with a long list of diseases, common and rare, when discussing malabsorption, whether one uses physiological criteria (i.e., carbohydrate malabsorption, amino acid transport defects, structural abnormalities), age of onset (neonatal, perinatal, etc.), etiologic factors (gluten sensitivity, parasite infestation, etc.), or even stool characteristics (fatty, watery). In practice, several factors contribute to the malabsorption simultaneously, and in most cases, especially if malnutrition complicates the picture, it is difficult to separate primary causes from secondary consequences.

The key to a successful evaluation of the patient with malabsorption is the systematic application of the knowledge of physiology and careful (and often painstaking) history taking. Examination of the stool, as described in Chapter 3, will also provide valuable information. The severity of symptoms and the impact on nutritional status and hydration will determine the urgency with which evaluation needs to proceed.

## PRESENTING SYMPTOMS

Early onset of diarrhea and failure to gain weight usually point to a brush border enzyme defect or to a defect of sugar transport. In these cases, removal of the offending carbohydrate can be lifesaving. Indispensable for the evaluation of carbohydrate malabsorption is familiarity with the composition of infant formulas. In other instances, onset is insidious, and diarrhea might not even be apparent. Steatorrhea can occur with few daily bowel movements while in a few children, apparent constipation is occasionally described. The bulkiness, smell, and fatness of the stool will provide important clues about possible underlying abnormalities in the digestion and absorption of foodstuffs.

Malabsorption should be suspected when there is:

- Failure to thrive
- Abdominal distention
- Excessive flatus
- Abnormal stools
- Bleeding diathesis
- Bone abnormalities (fractures, rickets)
- Skin manifestations of nutritional deficiencies.

The importance of regular monitoring of weight and height gains was stressed in Chapter 2, and should result in a full evaluation whenever the cause is not constitutional or insufficient caloric intake.

Tests for measuring suspected fat or carbohydrate intolerance are generally available, and many can be carried out by the practitioner in the office and even by the bedside. See also Chapter 3 for methods of investigation.

## ANATOMIC OR STRUCTURAL DISORDERS

Anatomic abnormalities resulting in malabsorption will present in most cases in the neonatal period:

- Intestinal atresia or stenosis
- Intestinal duplications
- Rotation abnormalities with volvulus and bowel loss (short bowel syndrome)

• Vascular/infectious (necrotizing enterocolitis)
• Lymphatic drainage anomalies (lymphangiectasia).

In later years, the same end result can follow extensive surgery for trauma, inflammatory bowel disease, or as a complication of radiation therapy to the abdominal organs.

## FUNCTIONAL CONSIDERATIONS

Functional integrity of the intestine depends on smooth integration of a great number of factors, including:

• Gastric acidity
• Secretory immunoglobulins
• Humoral and cell-mediated immune processing
• Prostaglandins
• Protective effects of glycoproteins in mucus
• Peristalsis.

Conditions affecting *immune competence* will often result in chronic diarrhea, recurrent gastrointestinal infections and infestations, mucosal damage, and malabsorption. Predisposition for certain parasite infections (e.g., *Giardia*, *Cryptosporidium*, atypical mycobacteria, etc.) are encountered in congenital and acquired immune deficiency syndromes (AIDS) and can become a major aspect of the patient's illness.

Early in life, diarrhea in the presence of thrombocytopenia should raise the possibility of Wiskott-Aldrich syndrome, while recurrent infections (pustular dermatitis, pneumonia, candidiasis) should result in a full evaluation of the humoral and cellular components of immunity.

Only a selected group of disorders will be discussed in the following section. These represent the most commonly encountered entities and offer an opportunity to review aspects of digestive physiology of practical interest.

### Disaccharidase Deficiencies

Brush border enzyme deficiencies can be congenital or more frequently, acquired, most commonly following infectious gastroenteritis or other damaging insults to the intestine (gluten-induced enteropathy, cow's protein sensitivity, giardiasis, etc.). A congenital defect involving the transport of glucose and galactose is extremely rare, but its identification in an infant presenting with severe diarrhea while on lactose or glucose feedings can be lifesaving.

Several enzymes possessing disaccharidase activity have been identified in protein extracts of the enterocyte. It is believed that only one *lactase* is of physiological significance in the hydrolysis of dietary lactose. The second lactase is located intracellularly, and does not appear to contribute to lactose digestion.

Several *maltases* have also been identified, responsible for the digestion of maltotriose released by amylase from plant starch. The molecular relation and sharing of active sites between sucrase and isomaltase is still of great interest to geneticists and biochemists, since deficiency of one enzyme is accompanied by abnormal activity of the second.

Once monosaccharides have been produced on the brush border, absorption depends on mechanisms coupled to energy-dependent, active sodium transport, probably requiring specific carrier proteins. Glucose and galactose are two monosaccharides known to be absorbed through this pathway, while fructose appears to be absorbed by a process of facilitated diffusion. Not all carbohydrate hydrolyzed by one enterocyte is absorbed in situ; rather, it is carried in the intestinal juice to be absorbed further downstream.

*Sucrase-isomaltase (S-I) deficiency* should be suspected when watery diarrhea follows introduction of foodstuffs containing sucrose (table sugar) (Table 4–1). The diarrhea is explosive and is accompanied by cramps and abdominal distention. All of these symptoms are typical of osmotic diarrhea, regardless of the carbohydrate involved. Treatment of S-I deficiency consists of strict avoidance of sucrose. Starch can still be consumed because most of its chemical make-up consists of amylose which generates glucose when digested by pancreatic amylase or by brush border glucoamylase at the 1–4 positions. When diagnosis is suspected on clinical grounds, a breath hydrogen test after a sucrose load or an abnormal sucrose tolerance test will help identify sucrose as the offending carbohydrate. Final diagnosis requires demonstration of abnormal sucrase-isomaltase activity in jejunal biopsy material in the presence of normal villus architecture.

## Lactose Intolerance

Lactase activity is markedly decreased following infectious gastroenteritis or injury to the mucosa caused by gluten or other sensitizing proteins. Recovery of full function might take months, since lactase is the last enzyme to return to normal. This secondary lactose intolerance has popularized the use of formulas containing sucrose or glucose polymers in children recovering from gastroenteritis. In addition, the potential of cow's protein to induce an allergic exposure in the infant with damaged intestinal mucosa has also encouraged the use of soy protein or protein hydrolyzates. There is evidence that implicates protein hypersensitivity in the prolonged course of diarrhea seen in some children, with progression to chronic forms of diarrhea.

TABLE 4–1.

Common Sucrose Sources

Table sugar (cane, beet, brown)
Jellies, marmalades
Syrup (maple, molasses)
Fruits
  Apple
  Apricot
  Orange
  Banana
  Melon
  Watermelon
  Pineapple
  Plums
  Fruit juice
Vegetables
  Peas
  Sweet potatoes
  Carrots
  Broccoli
  Cucumber
  Pumpkin
  Corn
Formulas containing sucrose
Condensed milk
Chocolate milk
Ice cream, sherbet
Sweetened cereals
Rice
Processed and cured meats, cold cuts

The presence of malabsorbed substrate in the intestinal lumen results in fluid shifts and osmotic diarrhea. Fermentation by bacteria contribute to the cramps and bloating. It seems prudent to withhold lactose, or at least to decrease its total intake, in children with gastroenteritis and for a period of 1 to 3 weeks thereafter if there is evidence of lactose intolerance (Table 4–2). An exception to this guideline is the recommended practice to continue breast feedings during acute gastroenteritis.

Ethnically related lactase deficiency is the most important reason for lactose intolerance in the general population. There is no satisfactory explanation to account for the eventual loss of enzyme activity after weaning. On a global scale, it is obvious that persistence of the ability to digest lactose is the exception rather than the rule. Mutation of a *regulatory gene* for lactase has been postulated to explain the delayed onset of hypolactasia in susceptible individuals. Continuing milk intake in populations known to become lactase deficient beyond the childhood years can affect the age of onset. Lactase does not behave as an inducible enzyme, but continued exposure to milk products can, to a certain degree, affect the regulatory gene.

The prevalence of lactose intolerance in the Caucasian population of the United States is about 20%, while in American Indians, Eskimos, Japanese, and Chinese, this number is close to 100%. The prevalence in the Scandinavian countries is low — 2%–15%. The age of onset of this ethnically associated lactase deficiency varies from early childhood to late teenage years. In the black American, symptomatic lactose intolerance increases after age 10 years.

### Diagnosis of Lactose Intolerance

Of the methods available for investigating the patient with suspected lactose intolerance, the breath hydrogen test is the least invasive and most sensitive (see Chapter 3). Clinical correlation at the time of the test is very important, since standard tolerance tests are usually performed with unphysiologic amounts of lactose (equivalent to drinking over two pints of milk at once!). Gastric emptying of lactose diluted in water is very different from gastric emptying of homogenized milk, and the rate of delivery of the carbohydrate to the mucosa is important in determining intolerance in those individuals with decreased lactase activity. Some will be able to tolerate small quantities of milk products when consumed together with other foods, especially if they contain fat.

Jejunal biopsy has been considered the "gold standard" for determining lactase activity, but the possibility of error caused by patchy lesions or sampling variations exists, and its use is limited to the more complicated clinical situations where morphological and functional assessment of the small intestine is needed.

Determination of blood glucose concentrations after an oral lactose tolerance test is fraught with many of the sources of inaccuracies mentioned above. Because it requires at least six blood drawings, it is not in widespread use and is being replaced by the breath hydrogen test in most medical centers.

TABLE 4–2.

Common Lactose Sources

---

Breast milk
Mammalian milks (whole, skim, low-fat)
Cream, ice cream, sherbet, pudding
Cheese
Yogurt
Creamed vegetables
Some processed mashed and fried potatoes
Unkosher meats and processed meat products
Many salad dressings, cream soups
Cookies, cakes, breads (unless marked "Parve")
  Zwieback, pasta
Some liqueurs, cordials

---

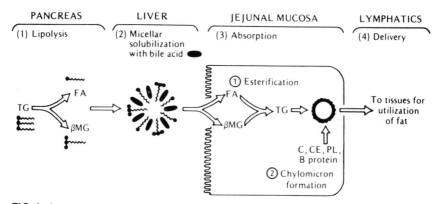

| PANCREAS | LIVER | JEJUNAL MUCOSA | LYMPHATICS |
|---|---|---|---|
| (1) Lipolysis | (2) Micellar solubilization with bile acid | (3) Absorption | (4) Delivery |

**FIG 4–1.**
Schematic of intestinal fat absorption showing the participation of pancreas, liver, and intestinal mucosal cell in fat absorption. (From Wilson FA, Dietschy JM: Differential diagnostic approach to clinical problems of malabsorption. *Gastroenterology* 1971; 61:911–931. Used by permission.)

## *Treatment*

Elimination of lactose-containing products has to be tailored to the degree of intolerance. In the most severe cases, the diet has to be strictly adhered to while other individuals will be able to indulge in some of their favorite cheeses and yogurts without suffering from cramps, gas, or diarrhea. Yogurt is an excellent source of calcium for children and adults with only moderate hypolactasia. Autodigestion of lactose by fermenting lactobacilli has been demonstrated in yogurt. Prehydrolyzed lactose is also found in special milks and milk products currently available in most supermarkets in the United States (LactAid).

For the child with severe intolerance, a calcium supplement 600 mg to 1,000 mg/day should be offered. Some convenient forms of calcium widely available include (1) calcium carbonate (i.e., Tums, Os-Cal, Cal-Sup, other tablets 250–1,000 mg, some with vitamin D); and (2) calcium glubionate (i.e., Neo-Cal-glucon syrup, 115 mg/5 cc).

## Fat Malabsorption

Bile salts are needed for micelle formation and emulsification of dietary lipid and fat-soluble vitamins (Fig 4–1). Triglycerides can then be attacked by pancreatic lipases prior to absorption of the free fatty acids and monoglycerides resulting from that hydrolysis.

Processing of lipids inside the enterocyte includes the resynthesis of triglycerides and their coating with lipoproteins prior to translocation into the lymphatics as chylomicrons. An efficient enterohepatic circulation returns 99% of bile acids back to the liver after reabsorption in the terminal ileum.

Interference with any of these processes can result in abnormal fat digestion and absorption, as seen in:

1. Cholestasis and severe liver disease
2. Lipase deficiency
3. Abetalipoproteinemia
4. Decreased intestinal absorptive area
   a. Short bowel syndrome
   b. Celiac disease
   c. Other enteropathies
   d. Giardiasis
5. Intestinal Lymphangiectasia
   a. Trauma to the lymphatic channels
6. Abnormal reabsorption of bile acids
   a. Congenital defect in transport mechanism
   b. Surgical loss
   c. Inflammation.

## STEATORRHEA

Recognition of steatorrhea is usually not difficult. The stools tend to be large and bulky because of their increased gas content (and tend to be light and float on the toilet water). A film of oil can be seen or oiliness to the touch noticed when changing diapers. The smell is typically foul.

Recognition of the child with *cholestasis* is not difficult if jaundice is present. In certain conditions, bile acid excretion is impaired with normal serum bilirubin concentrations. This is seen in some children with decreased number of intrahepatic bile ducts who are not jaundiced but have other biochemical signs of cholestasis (increased cholesterol, increased alkaline phosphatase, or 5' nucleotidase) and pruritus. Steatorrhea can be mild to severe.

*Isolated lipase deficiency* is rare, but isolated congenital deficiencies of amylase and trypsinogen have been described. Most commonly, pancreatic insufficiency is the result of cystic fibrosis and involves all zymogens. Pancreatic insufficiency is also part of *Schwachman's syndrome*, an inherited disease with abnormal bone marrow function (neutropenia, thrombocytopenia, anemia), eczema, and bone lesions (metaphyseal dysostosis). Pancreatic insufficiency results in severe failure to thrive, and neutropenia is responsible for the frequent and generalized infections (chronic purulent otitis, mastoiditis, meningitis). The primary defect in this syndrome remains unknown, but is different than cystic fibrosis. An important point of difference is that the sweat test is normal in Schwachman's syndrome.

*Abetalipoproteinemia* must be considered in the differential diagnosis of the child with failure to thrive, steatorrhea, and anemia. A biochemical clue is the presence of very low serum cholesterol concentrations (less than 50 mg/dl). The presence of acanthocytes (spiculated red blood cells) in the blood smear is also suggestive. The serum is not turbid after a fatty meal because of the basic inability to form chylomicrons and abnormal fat transport from the enterocyte. The diagnosis is confirmed by lipoprotein electrophoresis and with a jejunal biopsy which is characteristic and shows fat-laden villi. The progressive neurological deterioration (including retinitis pigmentosa, ataxia, ophthalmoplegia), until recently considered an inseparable part of the disease, has been found to be secondary to chronic vitamin E deficiency. Early diagnosis and institution of adequate vitamin E replacement will prevent or modify its development.

## CELIAC DISEASE

The term should not be used as a synonym for malabsorption syndrome or for the transient gluten intolerance that sometimes follows severe gastroenteritis or protein sensitivity (cow's milk, soy isolate).

Celiac disease is a *lifelong* intolerance to *gliadin*, a protein fraction present in the "germ" of wheat and rye glutens. Reaction to barley and oat gluten has not been consistent. Rice and corn are always tolerated.

The mechanism of gluten-mediated damage has not been fully clarified. A biochemical defect involving a mucosal peptidase or carbohydrase has been postulated but not conclusively proven. Immunological mechanisms seem to be partly responsible. Damage mediated by immune complex deposition in the lamina propria has also been demonstrated in certain cases. Increased production of serum IgA occurs during gluten exposure and usually returns to normal following strict diet therapy.

*Prevalence* is very high in West Ireland (1 in 300) while it is rare in Oriental and black populations. Association with HL-A phenotypes B-8 and DR W-3 has been documented.

The *pathological findings* in the jejunal biopsy explain the resulting malabsorption. In the untreated state, a flat intestinal mucosa is present throughout the duodenum and jejunum resulting in great loss of absorptive surface (Figs 4–2 and 4–3). The ileum is also sensitive to gluten, but usually preserves its villus structure. The mucosa is flat, but not really atrophic. There is enlargement of the crypts of Lieberkuhn, and rapid cell turnover. Intraepithelial lymphocytes are an important marker of celiac disease but their numbers do not always parallel activity or severity. After gluten withdrawal and mucosal recovery, damage caused by reexposure to gliadin can be patchy. This makes interpretation of the biopsy at the time of challenge difficult at times.

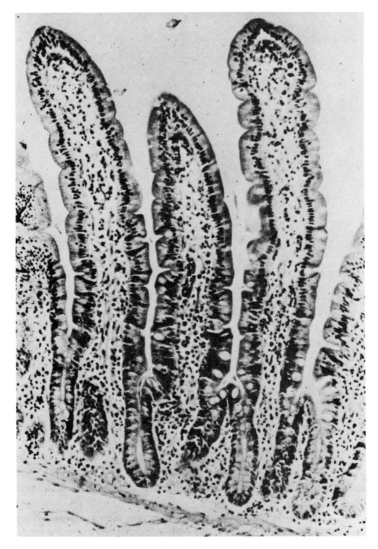

**FIG 4–2.**
Conventional histological appearance of normal jejunal mucosa. (×112). (From Creamer B: *The Small Intestine*. London, William Heinemann Medical Books, 1974. Used by permission.)

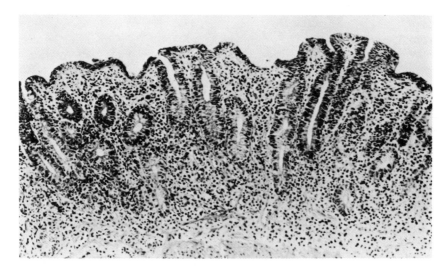

**FIG 4–3.**
Photomicrographs of a jejunal biopsy from a case of celiac disease showing profound mucosal atrophy. (×104). (From Creamer B: *The Small Intestine*. London, William Heinemann Medical Books, 1974. Used by permission.)

### Clinical Features

The age at onset generally tends to correspond to the time of introduction of gluten-containing cereals, but symptoms can be delayed by months or be very subtle. Celiac disease can present as failure to thrive, without an obvious gastrointestinal cause. Most common symptoms are:

- Diarrhea and weight loss
- Vomiting
- Abdominal distention
- Irritability and tiredness
- Abdominal pain
- Anorexia.

The personality changes can be striking. The child appears clingy and is easily upset, apathetic, and sometimes almost autistic. The improvement in behavior and disposition that occurs with the institution of the gluten-free diet is often dramatic and difficult to explain, since little morphological recovery is demonstrable at the time.

Some children will not have diarrhea, but rather constipation to the point of rectal prolapse. Voracious appetite is seen only in half of the children. When malnutrition is severe, edema, mucosal changes, muscle wasting, and anemia can be present at the time of diagnosis.

*Diagnosis*

*No child should be diagnosed as having celiac disease on the basis of a clinical response to gluten withdrawal.* A gluten-free diet for life is a major sacrifice for any child and his or her family. There should be no doubt that this recommendation is indicated.

After a child presents with failure to thrive and malabsorption is documented, a jejunal biopsy is indicated. This is especially the case if symptoms are temporally related to introduction of gluten-containing foods. Important information can be obtained from this low-risk procedure.

If the histology is compatible with celiac disease, a strict gluten-free diet should be instituted, probably for at least 2 years of good clinical response. At that time, a repeat biopsy should confirm the return of normal villus architecture.

A gluten challenge helps distinguish between transient gluten intolerance and celiac disease. Histological relapse can take 3 to 18 months to appear. For this reason, in the absence of clinical symptoms, the biopsy should be deferred 18 to 24 months to definitely confirm gluten tolerance. Reactions to reintroduction of gluten can be severe, sometimes producing shock (celiac crisis), so that the initial gluten challenge should be cautiously performed.

Reliable serum markers specific for celiac disease have not yet been developed, although there is obviously a great deal of interest in finding a noninvasive test able to obviate the need for jejunal biopsies. Antibodies to intestinal base membrane and reticulum have been found in some patients with untreated celiac disease and dermatitis herpetiformis, but validation of the findings and widespread application has not been carried out to everybody's satisfaction. Progress in immunopathology is hampered by the fact that the molecular defect(s) responsible for this disease remains unknown.

*Treatment*

Referral to a dietitian or nutritionist familiar with the management of celiac disease is very helpful. A variety of proprietary products is available in the better health food stores. National help groups are constantly updating their catalogs and exchanging recipes.*

Making the diet palatable and varied is important to recoup nutritional deficiencies many of these patients have at presentation. Initially, a lactose-free and cow's protein-free diet can be useful, since symptoms can resolve slowly if secondary lactose intolerance is present. In the most severe cases, a short course of oral prednisone can accelerate recovery.

---

* Gluten-Free Groups: Gluten Intolerance Group, P.O. Box 23053, Seattle, WA 98102-0353; Gluten-Free Products, Ener-G Foods, Inc., 6901 Fox Avenue South, P.O. Box 24723, Seattle, WA, 98124-0723, (206) 767–6660; American Celiac Society, 42 Gifford Avenue, Jersey City, NJ 07304, (201) 432–1207 or (201) 432–2986.

## Giardiasis

Infestation with this protozoon can range clinically from a totally asymptomatic carrier state to severe disease with diarrhea, malabsorption, and recurrent abdominal cramps. Giardiasis is by no means an exotic or tropical disease, and widespread epidemics can occur in crowded situations such as army barracks, summer camps, jails, or nurseries. Contamination of the water supply in rural and urban communities has been responsible for epidemics affecting thousands of individuals traveling to affected areas (Leningrad, Colorado, Kentucky, to name just a few of the most publicized incidents).

The trophozoite inhabits the upper small intestine, and chitin-enclosed cysts excreted in the stool can remain infective for months (Fig 4–4). Depending on the immune status of the host and other poorly understood factors, the parasite proliferates, actually attaching to the surface of the enterocyte by what appears under the electron microscope to be a "suction cup." Mechanical interference with nutrient transport and other effects on the microenvironment of the intestinal mucous layer have been postulated to explain the malabsorption. The parasite is known to metabolize bile salts, and interference with micelle formation is also possible. Patchy villus atrophy can result in secondary disaccharidase deficiencies. Bacterial overgrowth can be an additional complicating factor.

### Symptoms

Diarrhea can be indistinguishable from viral gastroenteritis, with similar symptoms but usually not accompanied by fever. Abdominal pain, nausea, loss of appetite, and passage of very foul stools can occur in the more severe cases with steatorrhea also present, and the stool can have the smell of rotten eggs (hydrogen sulfide).

### Diagnosis

Diagnosis requires a reliable parasitology laboratory. The cysts are not always detectable in the stool; special concentration techniques increase the yield. The stool can be collected in polyvinyl alcohol as a fixative, obviating the need to go to the lab with each fresh specimen. The yield of examining three separate stools is only about 60%.

More reliable is the sampling of duodenal contents, either with a fluoroscopically positioned suction tube or more simply, with a "string test." The patient swallows a small gelatin capsule containing a weighed cotton string. After 3 or 4 hours, the string is removed and the mucus adherent to it is squeezed onto a glass slide and examined under the light microscope. The typical trophozoites can be detected in over 75% of patients (Fig 4–5).

### Treatment

The three most commonly used medications for the eradication of *Giardia lamblia* are:

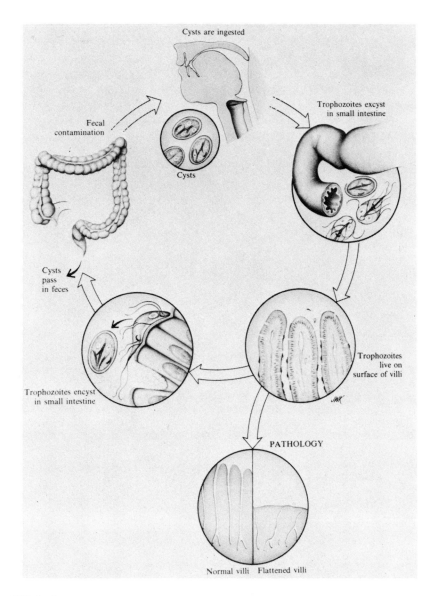

**FIG 4–4.**
Life cycle of the protozoan *Giardia lamblia*. The cyst is in the infective stage and is able to withstand adverse conditions of temperature, humidity, and exposure to chemicals. Excystation and encystation occur in the small intestine. (From Katz M, Despommier DD, Gwadz RW: *Parasitic Diseases*. New York, Springer-Verlag, 1982. Used by permission.)

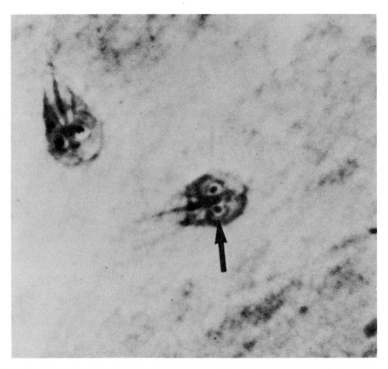

**FIG 4–5.**
Typical trophozoites of *Giardia lamblia*. The *arrow* points to two nuclei that contribute to the characteristic appearance. The six flagella are not clearly visible. (×800). (From Katz M, Despommier DD, Gwadz RW: *Parasitic Diseases*. New York, Springer-Verlag, 1982. Used by permission of the publisher and courtesy of Dr. D. Lindmark.)

1. Quinacrine hydrochloride (Atabrine)
   8 mg/kg/day for 5 days, maximum 300 mg/day
   Side effects: Nausea, headache, yellow discoloration of skin (clears after several weeks)
   Efficacy: 90%–95%. A second course might be necessary.
2. Metronidazole (Flagyl)
   40 mg/kg/day for 5 days
   Side effects: Nausea, vomiting, headache, metallic taste, alcohol ingestion contraindicated
               Neutropenia, usually not a problem in 5 days
               Tumorigenic effect in animals.
   Efficacy: 90%–95%

3. Furazolidone (Furoxone)
   About 5 mg/kg/day in 4 divided doses for 5 days
   Side effects: Nausea, vomiting, hemolysis in susceptible individuals
   Efficacy: 70%–75%.

Furoxone has the advantage of being the only preparation in liquid form and can be dosed more conveniently in the younger patients.

## BIBLIOGRAPHY

1. Berg NO, Borulf S, Jakoosson I, et al: How to approach the child suspected of malabsorption. *Acta Pediatr Scand* 1978; 67:403.
2. Gary GM: Carbohydrate digestion and absorption. *N Engl J Med* 1975; 292:1225–1230.
3. Riley JW, Glickman RM: Fat malsorption — Advances in our understanding. *Am J Med* 1979; 67:980–988.
4. Brandborg LL: Histologic diagnosis of diseases of malabsorption. *Am J Med* 1979; 67:999–1006.
5. Olsen WA: A pathophysiologic approach to diagnosis of malabsorption. *Am J Med* 1979; 67:1007–1013.
6. Falchuk ZM: Update on gluten-sensitive enteropathy. *Am J Med* 1979; 67:1085–1096.
7. Ament ME, Perera DR, Esther LJ: Sucrase-isomaltase deficiency: A frequently misdiagnosed disease. *J Pediatr* 1973; 83:721.
8. Mobassaleh M, Montgomery RK, Biller JA, et al: Development of carbohydrate absorption in the fetus and neonate. *Pediatrics* 1985; 75:160.
9. Lebenthal E, Lee PC, Heitlinger LA: Impact of development of the gastrointestinal tract on infant feeding. *J Pediatr* 1983; 102:1.
10. Watkins JB: Mechanism of fat absorption and the development of gastrointestinal function. *Pediatr Clin North Am* 1975; 22:721.
11. Tobey N, Yeh R, Huang TI, et al: Human intestinal brush border peptidases. *Gastroenterology* 1985; 88:913.

# 5

# Diarrhea

Diarrhea is an important illness in the pediatric age group; on a global scale, it is a major cause of infant mortality. Some of the factors responsible for the propensity for diarrheal disease in infancy are listed in Table 5–1.

For some infants, one bowel movement after each feeding is common, but to new parents, this often seems too frequent and causes concern. Reassurance and a brief explanation of the gastrocolic reflex is all that is needed in most cases. There should not be a water ring around the solid part of the stool, and one should be careful distinguishing between very large watery stools and stool that is mixed with urine. Serious diarrheal losses can be missed in some children with totally unformed bowel movements.

## DEFINITION AND PHYSIOLOGIC MECHANISMS

Diarrhea can be defined as an increase in the frequency or a decrease in the consistency of the stool. This definition implies a *change* from a habitual pattern and this concept is always important in the assessment of both diarrhea and constipation.

In more physiological terms, diarrhea can be defined as water malabsorption. Movement of water across the intestinal surface is passive and is coupled to the transport of electrolytes and other small molecules such as glucose or amino acids. Absorption takes place in an isotonic environment. Accumulation of un-

TABLE 5–1.

Factors Predisposing Children to
Diarrhea

Decreased immune defenses
  Specific immunoglobulins
  Opsonins
  Secretory IgA
Congenital anomalies
Enzyme deficiencies
  Lactase
  Sucrase-isomaltase
  Enterokinase deficiency
  Glucose-galactose malabsorption

absorbed solute in the lumen creates osmotic fluid shifts directed toward equalizing the solute concentrations between the lumen and the blood.

Movement of electrolytes in and out of the lumen is a complex process. Research into the mechanisms of fluid and electrolyte transport in the intestinal tract has provided new insights in the understanding of enterotoxin and tumor bile acid-induced diarrhea.

## ELECTROLYTE TRANSPORT

The understanding of electrolyte transport has been an area of intensive research in the past decade. Models of coupled-absorption, active, carrier-mediated and energy-dependent systems have been needed to explain some of the laboratory observations. In vitro studies, including work on cell preparations enriched for villi, crypts, or even basolateral membranes, have provided investigators with a wealth of data, sometimes unexplainable by current concepts. As the sophistication of the methodology increases, so does the complexity of the problem and its possible solutions.

In brief, sodium can be transported by passive solvent drag, or more importantly, by glucose or amino acid-stimulated active absorption. Active transport by electrogenic forces is more developed in the colon, where sodium can be reabsorbed even if the luminal concentration is as low as 30 mEq/L. The presence of sodium-hydrogen exchange mechanism in the jejunum has been demonstrated. This transport is enhanced by the presence of bicarbonate in the lumen. Glucose appears to stimulate the absorption of sodium in the jejunum, but the mechanism is not clear.

Chloride is also transported by active and passive processes. Most chloride is absorbed by a passive flow promoted by the electronegative charges of the mucosa. When the potential difference between the mucosa and the basal membrane increases (for example, when glucose stimulates sodium transport), more chloride is also absorbed. In exchange for bicarbonate, chloride is absorbed in the ileum and colon.

Active secretion of chloride, as can be shown to occur in diarrhea caused by enterotoxin, bile acids, or hormones, seems to take place in the crypts and is stimulated by increased concentrations of cyclic AMP or changes in intracellular calcium.

Potassium transport is believed to be passive, along electrochemical gradients, but the possibility of active secretion in the colon is still being investigated.

## STOOL COMPOSITION

High concentration of sodium is typical of stools in "secretory states," such as those that occur in enterotoxigenic diarrheas, or, classically, in the diarrhea induced by the cholera toxin. Sodium concentrations can approach 100–120 mEq/L, or close to the concentrations in serum. All the osmolality of the stool is accounted for by the concentration of sodium, potassium, and their anions. On the other hand, diarrhea caused by the osmotic influx of water into the lumen secondary to malabsorbed substrate (carbohydrate, unabsorbable salts) is low in sodium and higher in potassium (average: 20–40 mEq/L sodium, 30 mEq/L potassium).

## ABSORPTIVE CAPACITY OF THE INTESTINAL TRACT

The absorptive capacity of the small and large intestines is enormous. It is estimated that about 10 L of fluid is introduced in the lumen of an adult in the course of the day by salivary, pancreatic, biliary, gastric, and intestinal secretions. The amounts in a child are quantitatively smaller, but relative to the body weight, they are even larger, since the ratio of body weight to surface area is greater in the child than in the adult. In addition, the body composition of infants has larger proportions of water; therefore, fluid losses have a greater effect on homeostasis in the young child than in the adult. Some of the factors contributing to higher morbidity and mortality in children with diarrhea are listed in Table 5–2.

Of all those endogenous secretions, only 10% (or about 1.5 L in the adult) normally reach the colon. The jejunum has an efficiency for water reabsorption in the order of 50%, while the ileum reabsorbs about 75% of the volumes delivered from the jejunum and its intrinsic secretions. In the colon, all but 100 cc to 150 cc are reabsorbed, an efficiency of almost 90%. Any changes in the total volume of secretions results in a larger volume being delivered to the colon.

The colon can double its absorptive capabilities, but beyond that point, increased water will be lost in the stool. A small change in the water content of the stools will result in diarrhea.

## PATHOPHYSIOLOGY OF DIARRHEA

In assessing diarrhea, it is useful to think in physiological terms. In most cases, more than one of the mechanisms discussed will be at play, but identifying the primary mechanism narrows the range of diagnostic etiologies.

The most common mechanisms for diarrhea (Table 5–3) are discussed below.

### Secretory Diarrhea

The final common pathway to the production of secretory diarrhea is activation of cyclic nucleotides, mainly cAMP. It is difficult to be sure that the secretion is related to increased efflux and not to decreased influx, but functionally the *net flux* is what determines the end result, and defining secretory diarrhea in terms of the net flux is the only practical approach.

The hallmark of secretory diarrhea is its persistence while the patient is receiving nothing by mouth. This simple measure becomes an important diagnostic maneuver early in the evaluation and management.

The most important stimulants of adenyl cyclase are the toxins produced by certain *Vibrios* and *E. coli*, the products of bacterial deconjugation of bile acids or hydroxylation of certain short chain fatty acids (actually, very similar to octanoic acid, a chemical structure closely related to ricinoleic acid, the active agent in castor oil).

TABLE 5–2.

Factors Contributing to Increased Morbidity and Mortality From Diarrhea in Children

Large extracellular fluid compartment
Large intestinal surface to body-weight ratio
Increased metabolic demands
Decreased caloric reserves

TABLE 5–3.

Mechanisms of Diarrhea

Secretory
Osmotic
Abnormal motility
Obstruction to blood and lymph flow

Bacterial overgrowth can be responsible for generation of secretagogues in:

• Partial intestinal obstruction
• Blind loop syndrome
• Loss of the ileocecal valve
• Pancreatic insufficiency
• Short bowel syndrome.

The composition of the stool in the secretory diarrheas is characterized as mentioned, by neutral pH and high sodium concentration. A neutral pH is the result of acid neutralization by actively secreted bicarbonate.

In hypersecretory states such as produced by enterotoxins, the villus is generally well preserved. Provision of glucose-electrolyte solutions promotes sodium and water reabsorption, allowing successful oral rehydration (see below). Application of these principles in our day-to-day management of diarrhea has changed the composition of rehydrating solutions presently available.

## Osmotic Diarrhea

Whenever there is a nonabsorbable solute in the intestinal lumen, water will shift to attempt equilibration toward isotonicity. If normal motility is present, diarrhea results as the reabsorptive ability of the intestine is overloaded. Poorly absorbed solutes will have a similar but less prolonged effect. If the nonabsorbed solute can be metabolized by colonic bacteria, other manifestations will accompany the diarrhea, mainly bloating, nausea, and increased gas. Carbohydrate is fermented to organic acids, lowering stool pH to less than 5.0. Reducing substances can also frequently be detected. The stool will have a higher concentration of potassium than seen in secretory diarrheas, since the colon cannot conserve this cation, while some of the sodium is still effectively reabsorbed.

Two of the most common situations where osmotic mechanisms are primarily responsible for diarrhea include *carbohydrate intolerance* as seen in lactose malabsorption or during the use of *laxatives* such as magnesium salts or sodium sulfate. In contrast to secretory diarrhea, osmotic diarrhea ceases when the causative agent is discontinued, again an important diagnostic clue.

Agents that can be malabsorbed leading to an osmotic diarrhea are listed in Table 5–4.

The carbohydrate intolerance can be secondary to a loss of activity of brush border disaccharidases, most commonly secondary to acute gastroenteritis but also secondary to overloading of the intestinal absorptive function by substrate delivered too rapidly. The pylorus is the main controller of the rate of delivery of nutrients to the duodenum, so that conditions affecting the integrity of the pylorus can have noticeable effects on digestion and absorption. Pyloroplasty and vagotomy, antrectomy, or gastroduodenostomy are examples of conditions

TABLE 5–4.

Some Common Causes of
Osmotically Induced Diarrhea

Cathartics
    Magnesium hydroxide
    Magnesium citrate
    Sodium sulfate
Carbohydrates
    Lactose (glucose-galactose)
    Sucrose (glucose-fructose)
    Lactulose (fructose-galactose)
    Sorbitol (sweetener)

predisposing to the so-called "dumping syndrome," characterized by a shock-like state, hypoglycemia (reactive), pallor, and sweating following meals.

Decreased absorptive surface is seen in celiac disease, nontropical sprue, malabsorptive syndromes as seen in immunodeficiencies, or parasitic infestations with *Giardia lamblia* or *Strongyloides*.

In the management of liver failure, a nonabsorbable carbohydrate is used in an attempt to reduce ammonia production and its reabsorption in the colon. The sugar, a disaccharide composed of galactose and fructose (lactulose), cannot be digested by the brush border and results in osmotic diarrhea.

Lactulose also promotes the growth of lactobacillus species which are known to generate less ammonia. Fast transit time from the laxative effect of this medication also contributes to faster evacuation of nitrogenous substrate, which further decreases ammonia production. The use of lactulose is a good example of an osmotic diarrhea iatrogenically induced for therapeutic purposes. As was discussed in chapter 3, lactulose can be used to calculate intestinal transit times in conjunction with the measurement of breath hydrogen.

## Abnormal Motility

The role of motility and motility disorders in the pathogenesis of diarrhea is far from clear. The difficulties associated with accurate measurement of intestinal transit and with in vivo studies of innervation and motor conduction have hampered the study of this important area of intestinal physiology.

States of hypermotility and diarrhea can be seen during the use of cholinergic drugs or more rarely in endocrine disorders involving the parathyroid, the thyroid, or the adrenal glands. Hypomotility states also are associated with diarrhea. The mechanisms involved in the abnormal motility seen in diabetic intestinal paresis or in certain collagen vascular disorders (scleroderma, dermatomyositis, lupus) is not clear, but stasis and associated bacterial overgrowth plays a role and can sometimes be improved by judicious use of antibiotics.

*Evaluation of the Patient With Diarrhea*

One of the first considerations in the evaluation of the child with diarrhea is to assess the effect of the losses of fluid, electrolytes, and nutrients. If the diarrhea is of acute onset, dehydration, acid-base, and electrolyte imbalances will be the most immediate concerns.

The therapeutic approach will be determined by the age of the patient, the association with vomiting and other sources of excessive fluid losses (such as fever), and the presumptive etiology of the diarrhea.

Acute diarrhea is most often secondary to an infectious agent, viral or bacterial. Epidemiologic studies have shown the high frequency of rotavirus-induced diarrhea during the winter months in temperate climates. It is useful to know the pattern of infections in the community, since clusters will usually present and will allow recognition and more specific treatment, if necessary and possible.

The history is important in delineating the course of the diarrhea and its response to various changes in the diet, or its development after the introduction of specific foodstuffs or medications. The number of stools, their consistency, and presence of mucus or blood is useful in the differential diagnosis between bacterial and viral infections. Bulky, foul smelling stools are more consistent with steatorrhea and sometimes are the first indication of pancreatic insufficiency or cystic fibrosis.

Association with vomiting, fever, convulsions, rashes, and respiratory symptoms gives additional clinical clues of the etiology of the illness. History of travel, similar disease in other siblings, and family members or playmates should also be elicited.

*Laboratory Investigation*

In the evaluation of acute diarrhea, the most useful laboratory tests include (see also Chapter 3, "Investigation of GI Disorders"):

• Stool examination for pH, reducing substances, occult blood
• Urine analysis (cells, specific gravity)
• Serum electrolytes, BUN, and creatinine
• Stool for routine culture (*Shigella, Salmonella, Campylobacter*, and *Yersinia*)
• Stool for rotavirus detection.

In most protracted diarrhea, additional tests will become necessary and should be tailored to the individual patient, based on the information obtained during the medical history and initial screening laboratory investigations.

## Chronic Diarrhea

By convention, diarrhea lasting more than 3 weeks has been termed "chronic." Often, the initial damage to the intestine is produced by an infection, but the course of the illness does not follow the expected pattern of recovery. Factors responsible for more protracted diarrhea are multiple and involve many of the mechanisms previously discussed. To further complicate the clinical picture, malnutrition results in secondary effects due to impaired protein and calorie homeostasis, hampering functional recovery. Motility changes, cell regeneration, and cell turnover are also impaired, enzyme maturation is compromised, and the patient becomes intolerant even to the most "elemental" formula.

Chronic diarrhea progresses sometimes to an "intractable" state. Mortality in this situation was as high as 75% before the development of parenteral alimentation. Intercurrent infections often proved fatal.

The same year that Avery and coworkers described the syndrome of chronic intractable diarrhea with its high mortality (1968), the first report appeared on the use of intravenous nutrition through a catheter placed in a central vein in an infant with severe short bowel syndrome. It soon became clear that the only way to prevent death from malnutrition in this population of seriously ill infants was through the reversal of their extreme catabolic state by the use of prolonged intravenous nutrition. In most cases, an etiology for the diarrhea is not found and it usually resolves slowly.

The differential diagnosis of prolonged diarrhea, is presented in Table 5–5.

**Formulas**

Familiarity with the most commonly used infant formulas is an invaluable tool to the pediatrician. Formula composition should be learned the same way that one learns about diuretics, cardiotonics, or antibiotics.

In many cases, formula changes can be used as a diagnostic maneuver, with a specific question in mind. The numerous formulas in the United States market provide the practitioner with a unique array of different protein, fat, and carbohydrate sources. Differences between some of the formulas involve the carbohydrate only or the protein only and thus can be switched to test the patient's tolerance for a given component.

In the hospitalized patient, continuous nasogastric (NG) feedings have been found to result in improved fluid and nutrient balance when compared to bolus oral or nasogastric intakes. A trial of NG feedings can often decrease the need for intravenous alimentation.

The most frequently used formulas and supplements are presented in Table 5–6, and are arranged by their composition: cow's protein-based, soy protein-based, lactose-free, sucrose-containing, hypoallergenic formulations, low-fat, medium chain triglyceride-containing, etc.

Carbohydrate-free modules are also available and allow introduction of progressive amounts of carbohydrate chosen by elimination of the poorly tolerated

TABLE 5–5.
Etiology of Chronic Diarrhea

| | |
|---|---|
| 1. Infection | 5. Other Enzyme Deficiencies |
|    *E. coli* |    Enterokinase |
|    *Yersinia enterocolitica* |    Trypsinogen |
|    *Giardia Lamblia* |    Congenital lipase |
|    Rotavirus | 6. Immune Deficiencies |
|    CMV |    Hypogamma globulinemia |
| 2. Carbohydrate Intolerance |    IgA deficiency |
|    Primary enzyme deficiencies |    Combined immunodeficiency |
|      Lactose intolerance |    Defective cellular immunity |
|        Familial | 7. Metabolic |
|        Congenital |    Abetalipoproteinemia |
|        Late-onset |    Wolman's disease (acid lipase deficiency) |
|      Glucose-galactose malabsorption |    Acrodermatitis enteropatica |
|      Postgastroenteritis |    Familial chloride diarrhea |
|      Associated with parasitic infections |    Hormonal tumors |
|      Immune disorders |      WDHA* (Verner-Morrison syndrome) |
|      Mucosal diseases |      APUD-oma† |
|        Lactose |      Ganglioneuroma-neuroblastoma |
|        Sucrose | 8. Anatomic Abnormalities |
|        Monosaccharide |    Hirschsprung's disease |
| 3. Gastrointestinal Allergies |    Malrotation |
|    Cow's milk protein |    Partial obstruction-stenosis |
|    Soy protein |    Blind loop syndrome |
|    Gluten |    Enteric fistula |
| 4. Pancreatic Insufficiency |    Short bowel |
|    Cystic fibrosis |    Pseudo-obstruction |
|    Schwachman's syndrome | |

* WDHA: Watery Diarrhea Hypochloremia Alkalosis.
† APUD: Amine Precursor Uptake (and) Decarboxylation.

TABLE 5–6.
Commonly Used Formulas for Infant Nutrition

| CATEGORY | PROTEIN SOURCE | CARBOHYDRATE | FAT | EXAMPLES (MANUFACTURER) |
|---|---|---|---|---|
| Cow's protein, "humanized," lactose-based Premature formulas | Cow's whey Cow protein | Lactose | Coconut oil Soy oil | Enfamil (Mead Johnson) Similac, Similac PM 60/ 40 (Ross) SMA, Preemie SMA (Wyeth) Similac Special Care (Ross) |
| Soy protein, | Soy isolate + | Corn syrup | Soy oil | Isomil (Ross) |

*(continued)*

TABLE 5–6.  *Continued*

| CATEGORY | PROTEIN SOURCE | CARBOHYDRATE | FAT | EXAMPLES (MANUFACTURER) |
|---|---|---|---|---|
| lactose-free | L-methionine | Solids | | Isomil-SF (sucrose-free)(Ross) |
| | | Sucrose | Coconut oil | ProSobee (Mead Johnson) Soyalac (Loma Linda) |
| Carbohydrate-free | | | | |
| Soy protein | Soy isolate | None | Soy oil Coconut oil | RCF (Ross) |
| Protein hydrolysate | Casein hydrolysate | None | MCT oil Corn oil | 3232 A (Mead Johnson) |
| Hypoallergenic, lactose-free | Casein hydrolysate | Sucrose, modified tapioca | Corn oil | Nutramigen (Mead Johnson) |
| | Casein hydrolysate + amino acids | Corn syrup, modified tapioca | Corn oil MCT oil | Pregestimil (Mead Johnson) |
| MCT-oil (useful in cholestasis or short bowel syndrome) | Casein | Corn syrup, sucrose, lactose trace | MCT oil Corn oil | Portagen (Mead Johnson) |

one. Carbohydrate-free formulas, as a general rule, should cautiously be used outside the hospital setting, since some carbohydrate needs to be provided to prevent ketosis. Once the right combination is found, parents can be taught to prepare the mixtures at home.

## ORAL REHYDRATION THERAPY

The use of oral rehydrating solutions in the management of childhood (and adult) diarrhea has changed the outlook for millions of patients around the world. Twenty years ago it was found that water and electrolyte reabsorption in the small intestine was dramatically affected by the presence in the lumen of monosaccharides and neutral amino acids such as glycine and alanine. Application of these scientific principles in the management of cholera was spectacular, and the need for intravenous fluid replacement was limited to the small minority of more seriously depleted victims. The active cotransport of sodium and glucose is the basis for the use of oral rehydrating solutions, since this mechanism remains intact in toxin-induced secretory diarrheas such as occurs in infections with *Vibrio cholerae* or enterotoxigenic *E. coli.*

A great deal of discussion has taken place since the World Health Organization (WHO) adopted an isotonic solution containing 90 mmole/L of $Na^+$, 20 mmole/L $K^+$, 80 mmole/L $Cl^-$, and 30 mmole/L bicarbonate. The glucose concentration was 111 mmole/L or 2 gm%. Because stool electrolytes in noncholera diarrhea are much lower, concerns about the risks of inducing hypernatremia with a high Na replacement solution were voiced following the WHO recommendations. A solution containing 45–60 mmole/L $Na^+$ was considered more suitable.

After years of extensive field experience, it is clear that the WHO formulation is adequate for initial hydration of moderate to severe deficits, but additional *free water* needs to be administered concurrently, usually one-third of the calculated deficits given after the initial 4 hours of rehydration. It is also clear that once rehydration and volume expansion have taken place, the kidney can effectively regulate sodium concentration, preventing serious hypernatremia in most cases.

As an example, an infant with mild (less than 5%) or moderate (6%–10%) dehydration would receive 100 cc/kg of WHO oral solution (90 mm/L $Na^+$) over the first 4 hours, and then another 50 cc/kg of water over the following 2 hours. In 6 hours, reevaluation determines whether rehydration is complete or whether another 6-hour cycle takes place, based now on the new weight. Less than 1% of patients will fail on this regimen and will require intravenous hydration. If dehydration is only mild, rehydration volumes are half of those described above, i.e., 50 cc/kg for the first 4 hours and 25 cc/kg of free water in the next 2 hours.

Initial work in hypernatremic dehydration suggests that if rehydration is spread over a longer period (12 hours rather than 6 hours), use of the WHO solution is also very effective and is accompanied by a decreased incidence of convulsions, a dreaded complication. In addition, hyponatremic dehydration can also be reliably corrected, usually in 24 hours, with the 90 mmole/L solution.

Despite the monosaccharide intolerance that has been shown to occur during rotavirus gastroenteritis, successful oral rehydration can be accomplished in most cases. The abnormal glucose transport occurs in areas of damaged mucosa and this damage is typically patchy, sparing sufficient cells with intact transport ability. Similarly, even in infections with enteroinvasive bacteria such as *Campylobacter* or *Shigella*, oral rehydration seems able to accomplish the major aims of restoring fluid and electrolyte homeostasis and of preventing the progression of moderate dehydration to circulatory collapse and acidosis.

Solutions with 45 to 75 mmole/L $Na^+$ are probably as appropriate for the prevention of dehydration soon after diarrhea has begun and also for stool replacement in cases of viral enteritis where electrolyte composition of the stool is closer to 50 than it is to 90 mmole/L stool.

In isotonic dehydration, controlled studies have shown comparable results using a 60 mmole/L solution, so the great advantage of a WHO-type solution is in the treatment of hypernatremic and hyponatremic dehydration.

The most common reasons for failure of oral rehydration are:

• Inability to keep up with the losses (large purge rates, as seen in cholera)
• Protracted vomiting
• Ileus
• Carbohydrate intolerance.

An important finding in the extensive clinical trials of oral rehydration therapy has been the rediscovery that early introduction of nutrients during the therapy for diarrheal illness is more beneficial than "bowel rest" or starvation. As early as 24 hours after the correction of deficits, formula or breast feedings can be introduced. Despite increased stool volumes, the intestine is able to absorb enough to maintain nutritional status preventing the deterioration so commonly seen in children affected with recurrent intestinal infections.

Exposure of the intestine to certain carbohydrates appear to stimulate growth of the gut mucosa. The presence of oligopeptides and amino acids in the lumen can promote $Na^+$ absorption through different transport systems, thus potentiating the rehydrating capacity of the bowel.

Starvation, on the other hand, results in diminished disaccharidase activity and in impaired electrolyte and nutrient absorption. If lactose intolerance is present, avoidance of this carbohydrate in the refeeding formula is advisable. Breast milk, despite containing lactose, seems to be well tolerated and can help provide additional protective factors in the form of specific secretory immunoglobulins and other cellular elements. In a minority of patients with severe acquired monosaccharide intolerance, continued ingestion of glucose or sucrose in the formula can result in further damage to the mucosa. The end result of this vicious cycle of diarrhea, malabsorption, and malnutrition and its consequences can be the picture of "intractable" diarrhea of infancy, as mentioned before.

Replenishment of losses and maintenance of fluid and electrolyte balance with oral rehydration solutions has a salutary effect on nutritional status. This is probably due to preservation of appetite and to the frequent advice and follow-up of the patients at the time of oral rehydration treatment.

## SUMMARY

Oral rehydration with a glucose/electrolyte solution has proven safe and effective in the management of most diarrheal illnesses in neonates, infants, children, and adults. If given early enough and in sufficient amounts, severe dehydration can be corrected and IV hydration avoided. Provision of free water when the WHO 90 mmole/L $Na^+$ solution used is needed. Correction of mild to moderate deficits can be accomplished in 6 to 12 hours. The volume offered orally is, in general, twice the calculated fluid deficit. Slower replacement in hypertonic dehydration diminishes the risk of convulsions. Early introduction of feedings is recommended to stimulate intestinal recovery and avoid nutritional deficits.

A minority of patients will fail all attempts at oral rehydration and will require intravenous fluids for correction of acidosis and fluid/electrolyte imbalances. In those cases, oral alimentation might be severely compromised for prolonged periods of time in which case parenteral nutrition can be lifesaving.

## BIBLIOGRAPHY

1. Gryboski JD: Chronic diarrhea. *Curr Probl Pediatr* 1979; 9:5–51.
2. Phillips SF: Diarrhea: A current view of the pathophysiology. *Gastroenterology* 1972; 63:495.
3 Steinhoff MCH: Rotavirus: The first five years. *Pediatrics* 1980; 96:611–622.
4 Hirschorn N: The treatment of acute diarrhea in children: An historical and physiological perspective. *Am J Clin Nutr* 1980; 33:637–663.
5 Winters RW: *Principles of Pediatric Fluid Therapy*, ed 2. Boston, Little, Brown & Co, 1982.
6. Gall GD, Hamilton RJ: Chronic diarrhea in childhood. A new look at an old problem. *Pediatr Clin North Am* 1974; 21(4):1001–1017.
7. Parfer P, Stroop S, Greene HL: A controlled comparison of continuous versus intermittent feeding in the treatment of infants with intestinal disease. *J Pediatr* 1981; 99(3):360–364.
8. Rosenberg AJ: Infectious diarrhea in the pediatric patient. Curr Concepts Gastroenterol 1983; Jan/Feb: 20–29.
9. Pickering LK: Evaluation of patients with acute infectious diarrhea. *Pediatr Infect Dis (Suppl)* 1985; S13–S18.
10. Avery GB, Villaviciencio O, Lilly JR, et al: Intractable diarrhea in early infancy. *Pediatrics* 1968; 41:712–722.
11. Lloyd-Still JD: Chronic diarrhoea of childhood and the misuse of elimination diets. *J Pediatr* 1979; 95:10.

# 6

# Food Allergy

Considering the complexities of the interaction between ingested foods and the intestinal mucosa, it is not surprising that reactions to foreign proteins and other chemicals are commonplace. The remarkable fact is the effectiveness of antigen processing and the development of tolerance in the majority of children by the time they are 1 year of age.

Because of the high number of symptoms usually ascribed to or blamed on food allergies, the pediatrician, more than ever, needs a practical approach to the problem, based on common sense and free of parental pressures. The value of having an open mind when taking a dietary history is most important, and a knowledge of "food families" and composition of frequently used commercial foodstuffs will be helpful in the medical detective work often needed to unravel the obscure histories presented by concerned or prejudiced parents (Table 6–1).

## MECHANISMS OF FOOD ALLERGY

Not all adverse reactions to foods are allergic in origin, and the term should be used more precisely to describe reactions mediated through immune mechanisms. Some of the identified mechanisms include:

- IgE-mediated hypersensitivity
- Immune complexes between antigens and IgG
- Cell-mediated, delayed type hypersensitivity.

## 60    Chapter 6

TABLE 6–1.
Common Food Families (Partial Listing)*

### Animal

| CRUSTACEA | PELECYPODA | CEPHALOPODA | OSTEICHTYES |
|---|---|---|---|
| Shrimp | Oyster | Octopus | Sardine |
| Crab | Clam | Squid | Trout |
| Lobster | Scallop | | Salmon |
| Crayfish | Abalone | | Whitefish |

### Vegetable

| | | | |
|---|---|---|---|
| Bromeliaceae | Gramineae | Leguminosae | Rutaceae |
| Pineapple | Barley | Kidney bean | Lemon |
| Chenopodiaceae | Corn | Lima bean | Grapefruit |
| Spinach | Oats | String bean | Orange |
| Compositae | Rye | Pea | Solanaceae |
| Lettuce | Wheat | Peanut | White potato |
| Cruciferae | Rice | Soybean | Chili pepper |
| Horseradish | Juglandaceae | Liliaceae | Tomato |
| Cabbage | English walnut | Garlic | Sterculiaceae |
| Mustard | Pecan | Onion | Chocolate |
| Cucurbitaceae | Lauraceae | Asparagus | Cola |
| Squash | Cinnamon | Palmaceae | Umbelliferae |
| Cantaloupe | Bay leaf | Coconut | Carrott |
| Watermelon | | Polygonaceae | Caraway seed |
| Cucumber | | Buckwheat | Dill |
| Drupaceae | | Pomaceae | Celery |
| Almond | | Apple | |
| Plum | | Pear | |
| Peach | | Rosaceae | |
| Apricot | | Strawberry | |
| Cherry | | | |

* From Metcalfe DD: Food hypersensitivity. *J Allergy Clin Immunol* 1984; 73:749. Used by permission.

The IgE-mediated reactions can be of extreme severity, producing anaphylactic shock after exposure to minute amounts of the offending antigen. Direct exposure to the GI tract mucosa is usually needed to trigger the reaction, but cases have been described in which inhalation of food being prepared or cooked can result in the same severe reaction. This type of reaction is mediated through mast cells in the intestinal mucosa, and both histamine and prostaglandins have been implicated in the allergic cascade. It is less clear that immune complexes (Arthus type II reaction) participate in allergies to food, but IgG does have the potential to form complexes in vitro when reacting with certain antigens.

Cell-mediated delayed hypersensitivity (Type IV) can be expressed via intraepithelial lymphocytes. In some patients with cow's protein allergy, it has been found that a subpopulation of the circulating lymphocytes is specifically inducible to release leukocyte migration inhibition factor. This is suggestive of a T cell-mediated mechanism homing on the enterocyte and causing cell damage.

The mucosa of the intestinal tract becomes progressively more effective in blocking out foreign proteins (Table 6–2). Absorption of macromolecules is more pronounced in infants and children, one reason why reactions to food are more prevalent in the younger years. Absorption is also enhanced by damage to the mucosa, such as that which occurs with severe gastroenteritis or during sensitization to one particular antigen. In pancreatic insufficiency, processing of proteins is impaired and more exposure to foreign antigens takes place. Once the damage has occurred, multiple allergies can develop from absorption of "innocent bystander" antigens.

TABLE 6–2.
Schematic Representation of Antigen Processing by the
Intestine

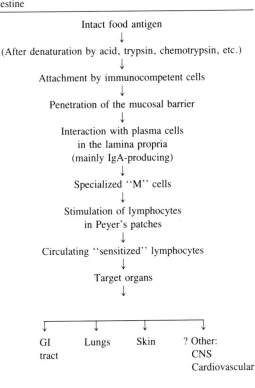

Intact food antigen
↓
(After denaturation by acid, trypsin, chemotrypsin, etc.)
↓
Attachment by immunocompetent cells
↓
Penetration of the mucosal barrier
↓
Interaction with plasma cells
in the lamina propria
(mainly IgA-producing)
↓
Specialized "M" cells
↓
Stimulation of lymphocytes
in Peyer's patches
↓
Circulating "sensitized" lymphocytes
↓
Target organs
↓

| GI tract | Lungs | Skin | ? Other: CNS Cardiovascular |
|----------|-------|------|-----------------------------|

## Protective Mechanisms

Keeping toxins and foreign antigens away is a complex process that involves immunologic and nonimmunologic components. The glycoproteins and glycolipids present in the mucus produced by ubiquitous glands throughout the GI tract, hydrolysis of proteins by gastric acid, and Kupffer cell engulfment of absorbed antigens all contribute to keeping the outside world away from the "self."

Immune protection is afforded locally by membrane epithelial cells (M cells) and intraepithelial B and T lymphocytes, part of the GALT, or gut-associated lymphoid tissue. The secretory IgA system is of particular importance in decreasing the invasiveness of bacteria. Dimeric IgA molecules attached by a "secretory piece" prior to their extrusion in the lumen are resistant to acid hydrolysis and effectively decrease bacterial and parasitic adhesiveness to the enterocyte. In conditions of selective IgA deficiency or generalized hypogammaglobulinemia, protracted gastrointestinal disease is often the presenting complaint and an important determinant of the patient's morbidity.

## Antigens in Food

Every food imaginable has been implicated in cases of abnormal reactions to ingestion. Whether the underlying mechanism is an allergic one or not cannot be determined in most cases, but from a practical standpoint, once the suspicion is raised that something in the diet is responsible for the patient's symptoms, our role is to narrow the range of possible allergens, establish the causal relationship, and prove it by a process of elimination and careful rechallenge.

Milk proteins are the best defined antigens and probably the most common factor in childhood food allergies.

When milk curdles, two major protein fractions are generated: the soluble whey and the precipitated casein. Caseins constitute about 80% of cow's milk protein compared to only 60% in human milk. Whey proteins are considered to be the most immunogenic, particularly the ones contained in the lactalbumin fraction: beta-lactoglobulin, alpha-lactalbumin, and serum albumin (Table 6–3). In addition to those proteins synthesized in the mammary gland of the cow, sensitization can occur to bovine serum proteins passively excreted in the milk. Similarly, human milk can contain foreign proteins circulating in the mother, and these are able to induce allergy even in the exclusively breast-fed infant (Table 6–4).

Interestingly, in view of the recent popularity of goat's milk, cross-reactivity with cow's milk proteins is frequent since they share antigenic similarities. Clinically, positive challenges to goat's milk have been reported in children with documented cow's milk allergy. Raw cow's milk has been shown to contain other substances potentially allergenic such as antibiotics, bacteria, and pesticides.

TABLE 6–3.
Protein Constituents of Cow's Milk

| CATEGORY | PERCENT |
| --- | --- |
| Caseins | 75%–85% |
| Whey | 10%–15% |
|   Alpha-lactalbumin* | 2%–5% |
|   β-lactoglobulin* | 7%–10% |
|   Albumin | 0.5%–1% |
|   Immunoglobulins | 1.5%–2.5% |

* Most commonly implicated in children with cow's protein allergy.

TABLE 6–4.
Other Allergens Occasionally Found in Cow's Milk

Bovine serum proteins
Penicillin and other antibiotics (streptomycin, tetracycline)
  Wheat
  Peanut (present in fodder)
  Cottonseed
  Insecticides
  Other adulterants

When milk is heated, some of its proteins are denatured, thus becoming less allergenic. Whey proteins are among the heat labile fractions, and some patients will tolerate milk that has been boiled. Caseins are stable at 100°C. Digestion of caseins with trypsin markedly reduces their antigenicity, and casein hydrolysates are commonly used in proprietary "hypoallergenic" formulas such as Nutramigen and Pregestimil (Mead-Johnson).

Other proteins commonly implicated in food allergy include ovalbumin (eggs), fish and shellfish, nuts, including chocolate (cocoa), yeast, and fruits from the rose (strawberries and other berries), citrus, and plum families. Soy has been used as a hypoallergenic protein source, but as many as 30% of patients with cow's protein allergy have also shown reactions to soy, and it appears to be an important cause of food allergy in children since it is so frequently prescribed as a substitute of choice when formula intolerance is suspected. The better tolerance of soy-based formulas after gastroenteritis is more likely to be related to its being lactose-free rather than to their having a different protein source.

## Clinical Aspects of Food Allergy

The most common manifestations of milk allergy are diarrhea, vomiting, and abdominal pains. A third of the patients will have allergic rhinitis and atopic dermatitis (Table 6–5).

Less than 15% will present with anaphylaxis. Half of the patients will have more than one symptom. If the intestinal damage is severe enough, steatorrhea, protein-losing enteropathy, occult or frank GI bleeding, and iron deficiency anemia can develop over a period of weeks or months, resulting in poor weight gain and malnutrition.

Symptoms can occur immediately following ingestion of the offending antigen, or slowly over a period of days. These two different patterns make the interpretation of food challenges difficult at times, since exposure has to be continued for at least 48 hours, if not more, in order to determine a cause and effect relationship.

Other respiratory symptoms include asthma, chronic cough, and signs of bronchial or small airway congestion. The association of pulmonary infiltrates from recurrent pneumonia, hemoptysis, and wheezing has been described in a few cases with the so-called *milk-induced syndrome with pulmonary disease* (Heiner). In addition, those patients exhibited iron deficiency anemia, eosinophilia, and failure to thrive. Milk-induced *hemosiderosis*, recurrent pneumonia, hemoptysis, and anemia are also found in some children, and this diagnosis is strongly suggested by the presence of iron-laden macrophages in the sputum or gastric washings.

Skin manifestations can occur in 50%–75% of infants with cow's milk allergy. Eczema or atopic dermatitis are most commonly encountered, urticaria less frequently so. Local reactions in the lips and oral mucosa, perianal irritation, and other rashes occurring after food ingestion have been observed.

TABLE 6–5.
Well Established Clinical Manifestations of Food Allergy

| SYSTEM | EXPRESSION |
|---|---|
| GI tract | Vomiting |
| | Diarrhea |
| | GI bleeding |
| | Protein losing enteropathy |
| | Bloating |
| | Anorexia |
| | Failure to thrive |
| Pulmonary | Rhinitis |
| | Wheezing, sneezing |
| | Hemoptysis |
| | Hemosiderosis |
| Skin | Urticaria |
| | Eczema |
| | Fixed eruptions |
| | Diaper rash |
| | Perioral edema, blisters |

More controversial and difficult to prove are behavioral and psychological reactions interpreted by some as allergic manifestations in the central nervous system. The *allergic tension fatigue syndrome*, as it has been called, includes such nonspecific symptoms as inability to concentrate, restlessness, depression, learning difficulties, headaches, tiredness, myalgias, growing pains, and respiratory congestion. Iron deficiency anemia can also be present. Interestingly, a similar constellation of psychiatric and physiologic features is present in the untreated child with gluten-sensitive enteropathy, and the response to a gluten-free diet can be as dramatic as that seen in the allergic tension fatigue syndrome when a successful elimination diet is instituted.

### Differential Diagnosis

*Infectious gastroenteritis* can initially mimic all the symptoms of food intolerance. The acute onset, presence of fever, epidemiologic considerations, and clinical course will usually help in the diagnosis. Parasitic and protozoan infestation, on the other hand, can present insidiously over many weeks and months. Abdominal distention, diarrhea, steatorrhea, anorexia, and worsening of symptoms in relation to meals can be difficult to distinguish, and stool examination or a "string test" to sample duodenal contents can be very helpful. *Carbohydrate intolerance* (lactose, sucrose, or, more infrequently, glucose-galactose malabsorption), whether primary or secondary to villus damage, should be considered in every case of food and formula intolerance. Symptoms associated with rapid intestinal transit, osmotic diarrhea, and fermentation of malabsorbed substrate are often clinically indistinguishable from immunologically mediated food allergies. *Direct pharmacological toxicity* to medications, food additives, or contaminants needs also to be considered. Vasoactive substances found in certain cheeses, caffeine, and other methylxanthines found in drinks and many antibiotics can affect the GI tract directly and suggest allergy. *Celiac disease*, a specific intolerance to gliadin, a component of gluten found in wheat, rye, and other cereals, can present with gastrointestinal symptoms suggestive of food allergy (see Chapter 4). Abdominal distention and loose bowel movements can be prominent. Some patients will have only one or two stools a day, but their description and analysis confirms steatorrhea. Failure to thrive, muscle wasting, and iron and folic acid deficiencies can be part of the full-blown celiac syndrome or develop secondary to other *protein allergy enteropathies*. Occult blood loss detectable by benzidine testing of the stool (Hemoccult) can result from microscopic or obvious colitis triggered by cow's milk allergy.

The differential diagnosis of *colitis* in a young child includes, in addition to the idiopathic chronic ulcerative form, infections with enteropathogens such as *Salmonella, Campylobacter, Shigella*, or *Yersinia*. Involvement of the colon by rotavirus can also occur. The presence of pulmonary symptoms suggestive of hypersensitivity, wheezing, recurrent bronchitis or cough, and gastrointestinal complaints worsened by food ingestion should always prompt a consideration of *cystic fibrosis*. At times, pulmonary symptoms can be minimal, and diarrhea or steatorrhea be more obvious. Interestingly, there is evidence to suggest that patients with pancreatic insufficiency have a higher incidence of food allergies, probably related to abnormal antigen processing in the intestine.

### Nonspecific Diarrhea of Childhood

Probably one of the most common causes of loose stools in children under age 4 years who otherwise are well and thriving is the interesting syndrome of chronic nonspecific diarrhea of childhood, sometimes also called the "irritable bowel syndrome." It is usually a diagnosis of exclusion, but the clinical picture is characteristic. Diarrhea usually appears around the first birthday and clears gradually by age 3–4 years. Stools tend to be mucoid, large, and running out of the diaper, and visible vegetable fibers are common (and not abnormal considering that fiber is, by definition, indigestible). Four to six movements a day are commonplace.

Positive family histories of functional intestinal disorders are frequent. Parents tend to be educated and extremely conscientious about charting stool number and dietary manipulations. Concern is evident in their faces and reactions.

Major considerations in the differential diagnosis include:

• Carbohydrate intolerance
• Postgastroenteritis-diarrhea
• Parasitic infestations
• Protein allergy
• Celiac disease
• Cystic fibrosis
• Intestinal lymphangiectasia.

In most of these children, simple manipulation of the diet and reduction of total fluid intake (especially of high carbohydrate drinks and fruit juices) are helpful. A low-fat diet is also a common finding among this group of children, either because of the parents' beliefs that such a diet is more healthful, or because their physicians have instituted restricted intakes for prolonged periods of time.

Often, a return to a more normal diet and restriction of fluids can result in a dramatic and welcomed change in the stool pattern. Toilet training improves the diarrhea. A motility disorder — perhaps mediated by prostaglandins — has been postulated because of the clinical response to aspirin, although few people advocate the treatment of nonspecific diarrhea with aspirin. Bile salt stimulated secretion in the colon has been implicated in a recent study involving a small number of children.

## Diagnosis

The diagnosis of food allergy is made on the basis of the clinical history and the response to a carefully designed elimination diet. Overdiagnosis is common, and this results in unfair limitations to the patients and their families. Ascribing a host of complaints to food allergy does not always result in their resolution. The bewilderment and frustration of parents trying to understand what they are doing wrong with their child's feedings is usually avoidable if the problem is approached with an open attitude from the beginning. There is no point in being dogmatic about the relation of suspected allergies and common gastrointestinal symptoms such as gas, green stools, colic, or regurgitation.

The younger the child, the easier it is to sort out a possible connection between ingested food and symptoms. The history should focus on the specific components of the intake, their amounts, frequency, and associated responses. A thorough knowledge of the composition of infant formulas and baby foods is necessary to properly evaluate a suspicion of allergy. A common mistake is to change formulas without realizing that all that has been changed is the name of the manufacturer. One should become familiar with a number of formulas and know their protein, carbohydrate, and fat composition. Only with this in hand will it be possible to thread the murky waters of elimination and substitution diets. Being able to change formulas to change just one component of the intake is a powerful diagnostic tool, and the pediatrician can then take full advantage of the large variety of proprietary formulas available nowadays (see Chapter 3).

Associated features to be elicited in the evaluation are other pulmonary, dermatological, or immunological manifestations of atopy. A family history, if reliable, is also useful. More often, evidence of milk and other allergies and even "celiac disease" in other family members (close and distant) is totally based on hearsay and is more confusing than helpful.

Asking the parents to keep a food diary can be revealing and gives them an opportunity to be objective, concentrating on the reporting rather than on the interpretation of symptoms. At times, a clear correlation will be evident from the diary, and a lack of correlation will also be important information. Diaries should be kept for a full week or 10 days since, in certain instances, ingestion of the inciting food is not frequent enough to allow detection.

### Laboratory Tests

Laboratory investigations can offer support to a tentative diagnosis of allergic mediated symptoms, but negative results do not rule out food allergy. Peripheral eosinophilia (absolute eosinophil count greater than 400/cu mm) is suggestive of allergy, but not necessarily of food allergy. In fact, neutrophilia was seen more commonly during challenge in milk-allergic children. Eosinophilic debris can be detected in the stool, the so-called Charcot-Leyden crystals, or in gastric mucus and other secretions of children who are food allergic. Serum immunoglobulins can show a diffuse or specific pattern of abnormality. Selective IgA deficiency is commonly associated with gastrointestinal symptoms including allergy. Elevation of the IgE fraction is highly suggestive of a hypersensitivity-mediated mechanism. Parasitic infestation and pulmonary allergies can elevate the serum IgE.

More sophisticated tests of food allergy have been developed in recent years; none is fail-proof and a negative test does not rule out clinical disease. The radioallergosorbent (RAST) technique allows identification of IgE antibodies against specific antigens located in specially treated paper discs. The test is expensive and requires a reliable laboratory. It is precise and reproducible, but antigens need to be standardized. The RAST technique is useful for screening highly allergic patients in whom previous reaction have been worrisome or life threatening. In patients with extensive atopic dermatitis where skin scratch or prick tests are not feasible or recommended, the RAST test offers a valuable alternative when performed by a reliable allergist. New antibodies to IgG-mediated allergic reactions will expand the usefulness of this test. Other in vitro tests for food allergy, such as precipitation and agglutination tests or identification of antibodies in the stool (coproantibodies), have not gained widespread use because of their lack of specificity and sensitivity and the problems associated with the processing of fresh stool needed for some of the tests.

## Management

Elimination of the suspected protein is instituted when a reasonable working hypothesis is formulated in the individual patient. Based on the history, review of food diaries, and an intelligent guess, the diet is modified either singly or by elimination of several high-risk food groups. It is most important to be familiar with the many ways in which milk, egg, or wheat products are hidden in commonly used foodstuffs. Processed meats (unless they are kosher) will usually contain milk as fillers. The same applies to prepared soups, cereals and pasta, baked goods, pudding, and of course, ice cream. Chocolate contains milk and egg proteins and is one item to avoid in any highly sensitive patient. Other highly allergenic products include corn, nuts and legumes (including soy), fish, and cola.

The elimination diet should be continued for at least 3 weeks before deciding whether it has been useful or not. Comparison of symptom scores, based on the diaries, is a way of semiquantitating the response. After symptoms have improved or subsided, reintroduction of new foods is made slowly, one at a time every week or two. If the patient is confirmed milk allergic, no challenge should be made for at least 6 months. Based on the initial presentation and severity of the intolerance, this period should be extended to a year or two. As the child grows, tolerance develops for many foreign proteins, and only a minority of milk-allergic children will remain so after the toddler years. On the other hand, other patients might develop allergies later in life. The mechanism for this phenomenon is not fully understood.

As mentioned before, many proteins are heat-labile, and denaturation by cooking will make them less allergenic. It is good practice to avoid the ingestion of uncooked food such as beef or fish in highly allergic individuals.

If one concludes at the end of the investigation that wheat-related symptoms are highly probable and if the patient has the signs of malabsorption syndrome ( see Chapter 4 ), arrangements should be made for consultation with a gastroenterologist. A jejunal biopsy is necessary to rule out celiac disease. More harm is done by empirically placing a patient on a longstanding gluten-free diet than by documenting villus atrophy prior to the institution of such a restrictive diet. Celiac disease is a lifelong diagnosis that should not be made on the basis of the clinical response alone, since the implications of not following a strict gluten-free diet for life are not totally clear. There are reports of increased intestinal neoplasms in untreated celiac patients, and although the evidence is not firm, it is known that gluten intolerance can be well established with total or subtotal villus atrophy but with few clinical signs or symptoms.

The nutritional and immunologic consequences of a damaged gut barrier are only beginning to be fully appreciated. Until then, it seems prudent to continue a gluten-free diet for life once the diagnosis of gluten-induced enteropathy has been confirmed by rechallenge after normalcy was demonstrated while being on a strict gluten-free diet. Unfortunately, there are no shortcuts when it comes to the diagnosis and management of celiac disease.

## BIBLIOGRAPHY

1. Bahna Sami L, Heiner DC: *Allergies to Milk.* New York, Grune & Stratton, 1980.
2. Speer F: *Food Allergy*, ed 2. Littleton, Mass, John Wright PSG, Inc, 1983.
3. Crawford LV, Herrod HG: Allergy diets for infants and children. *Curr Prob Pediatr* 1981; 9:12.
4. Stern M, Walker AW: Food allergy and intolerance. *Pediatr Clin North Am* 1985; 32(2):471–492.
5. Metcalfe DD: Food hypersensitivity. *J Allergy Clin Immunol* 1984; 73:749–762.
6. Lesof MH: Food intolerance and allergy — A review. *Q J Med*, New Series LII. 1983; 206:111–119.
7. Bock AS: Food sensitivity — A critical review and practical approach. *Am J Dis Child* 1980; 134:973–982.
8. McCarthy EP, Frick OL: Food sensitivity: Keys to diagnosis. *J Pediatr* 1983; 102:645–652.
9. Weinberg EG, Tuchinder M. Allergic tension fatigue syndrome. *Ann Allergy* 1973; 31:209.
10. Grieco MH. Controversial practices in allergy. *JAMA* 1982; 247:3106.

11. Stare FJ, Whelen EM, Sheridan M. Diet and hyperactivity: Is there a relationship? *Pediatrics* 1980; 66:521.
12. Lothe L, Lindberg T, Jakobson I. Cow's milk formula as a cause of infantile colic: A double blind study. *Pediatrics* 1982; 70:7.
13. Powell GK. Milk and soy-induced enterocolitis: clinical features and standardization of challenge. *J Pediatr* 1978; 93:553.

# 7

# Intestinal Gas

Hardly a day passes in the life of a pediatrician without mention of gas or symptoms ascribed to it. One of the first things a parent learns is to help the baby burp, and at times great difficulties seem to be encountered in this physiological process. Passage of flatus, cramps, colic, irritability, and apparent pain can easily be blamed on "trapped" gas or to excessive amounts of gas. So much distress is caused by an infant's crying that everything imaginable will be tried in an attempt to soothe the infant, mainly by providing an outlet for retained gas (thermometers, suppositories, etc.). Surface agents such as simethicone are commonly prescribed for the management of the colicky infant, despite the fact that their effectiveness has never been proven in controlled clinical experience.

It is useful to review the composition of intestinal gas, the underlying metabolic pathways of its production, and a sensible way to approach the problem when the excessive gas results from easily identifiable mechanisms.

## SOURCES OF INTESTINAL GAS

The two main sources for gas found in the intestinal tract are swallowed air and gas produced by intestinal bacteria (usually colonic) by fermentation of malabsorbed substrate. The three most common gases endogenously produced in the human intestine are hydrogen, methane, and carbon dioxide, comprising close to 99% of intestinal gases. All three of them are nonodorous, so the particular smell of flatus is caused by minute amounts of a large variety of trace gases (more than 200 have been identified). Volatile short chain fatty acids, scatols, hydrogen sulfide, and mercaptans are just a few, and interestingly, accumulation of some of these gases may reflect specific metabolic derangements with detectable pulmonary clearance. In hepatic failure, for example, mercaptans produced by colonic bacteria have been identified as contributors to the typical "fetor hepaticus." Similarly, volatile compounds generated in the colon and expired through the lungs will sometimes be responsible for nondental halitosis.

Methane is only produced by one third of the population, and the characteristic is genetically determined, although in some cases of institutionalized children, this capacity seemed acquired. It is not clear whether the trait results in a particular bacterial ecology which generates methane or is rather the inability to properly process normally produced gas.

Hydrogen is only produced in the human by bacterial metabolism. Malabsorbed carbohydrate is the major source. Lactose intolerance results in large volumes of hydrogen production. Complex carbohydrates such as those found in some flatulent vegetables (beans, asparagus, brussel sprouts, mushrooms, cauliflower, and cabbage, among many others) are also consistent sources of hydrogen. In fact, the "flatulence factor" present in beans was traced to two nonabsorbable carbohydrates — stachyose and raffinose. Beans without these carbohydrates can be produced by genetic hybridization techniques, a great addition to the diet of astronauts who until then had to be content with the problem of excessive gas in a weightless environment.

In addition to the carbon dioxide generated in the colon by bacteria, some is generated by the neutralization of gastric hydrochloric acid by pancreatic and biliary bicarbonate. Most of the $CO_2$ produced in the duodenum gets absorbed into the circulation and never reaches the colon. The partial pressure of $CO_2$ in the portal circulation is much lower than in the duodenum, favoring prompt absorption as this gas is generated. Conversely, because the partial pressure of $CO_2$ is greater in the blood than in the intestinal lumen, some of this gas will also diffuse passively. Quantitatively, this mechanism contributes little to flatus volume and composition.

The presence of carbonic anhydrase in the intestinal mucosa allows rapid metabolism of carbon dioxide. Since $CO_2$ is used to insufflate the colon at the time of procedures generating electrical sparks, the disappearance of this gas can result in a composition of gases potentially explosive (hydrogen and methane). Such accidents have been described. Carbon dioxide will not ignite; ignition is a dangerous possibility when methane and hydrogen are the prevailing gases.

If identification of air passed per rectum is needed, as may be the case in some extreme and bizarre situations, chromatography can immediately reveal the presence of a high concentration of nitrogen, confirming the aerophagic source of the problem.

## CLINICAL EXPRESSIONS OF INTESTINAL GAS

For practical purposes, gas can manifest as:

• Burping or belching
• Abdominal distention and pain
• Borborygmi
• Flatulence.

During the process of swallowing, air is gulped down with the food, sometimes in great amounts, depending on the degree of esophageal air trapping which occurs when inspiration takes place with a closed glottis. Chewing, crying, nervousness, talking, and drinking through a straw can exaggerate aerophagy.

Esophageal trapping of air can explain certain instances of *recurrent, noisy belching*. This occurs most commonly in older children and adolescents and can be an expression of a psychosomatic disorder or a technique learned accidentally and later turned into a habit expressing conscious or subconscious needs. This form of belching can be very disruptive to the family's social life, despite the attempts to excuse it as an involuntary phenomenon resulting from a "stomach problem." Management can be simple if the patient is ready to let go of the symptom, but very difficult if it reflects deeper and more complex derangements ("eructeo nervosa"). Sometimes, explaining to the family and the child the mechanism of aerophagy and stressing the fact that no air is actually produced in the stomach can be helpful. There is no way that a noisy, explosive release of air can take place a few minutes after another, unless that air is being swallowed. A conscious effort and prevention of inspiration on a closed glottis can rapidly eliminate the problem.

Belching is an expected experience after consuming carbonated drinks. The solubility of $CO_2$ decreases as the liquid warms up to body temperature and gas is further released by the churning action of the stomach contractions. As the gas bubble rises to the top, it encounters the gastroesophageal junction when the patient is in the sitting or standing position, and makes its way up to the outside world when the GE junction relaxes during a swallow. The relative position of the GE junction and the fundus in infants tends to favor burping while on the supine position. In adults, gas is more easily eructated when the patient is prone.

Abdominal distention can be the first expression of intestinal obstruction. Minutes after the first cry, gas can be found in the small intestine, and in one hour it usually reaches the colon. In the presence of intestinal stenosis or atresia, the gas accumulates, producing distention, often accompanied by bilious vomiting.

In the absence of obstruction, distention can most commonly result from gastric or colonic distention. Some infants will swallow a great deal of air when irritable and screaming.

Borborygmi are the "rumbles" caused by the propulsion of intestinal contents in the presence of gas distending the bowel loops. At times the sounds are embarrassingly loud or a source of concern. In most cases, borborygmi are a normal occurrence, especially after ingesting large volumes of fluids or during hunger pangs, and should be explained in simple physiological terms. In conditions of partial or total intestinal obstruction, borborygmi reflect the accumulation of gas and fluid in distended small intestinal segments. Peristalsis can be high pitched and hyperactive, frequently accompanied by crampy abdominal pains.

## AN APPROACH TO FLATULENCE

Notwithstanding the great deal of bewilderment generated by matters of intestinal gas, effective control is possible in a majority of patients. In the colicky infant, passage of flatus is most often an expected consequence of excessive crying, aerophagia, and vigorous abdominal wall muscle contractions. Undoubtedly, distention by "trapped" gas contributes to the painful crisis and help can often be provided by measures that favor expulsion of colonic gas.

Dietary control of excessive gas production involves elimination of flatulent foodstuffs. Limiting their intake to a few items makes the process of elimination and re-challenge easier to interpret. Among the cereals, rice has been found to be particularly well tolerated and results in less hydrogen production. Similarly, dilute orange juice is less likely to result in fermentation and gastrointestinal symptoms than grape juice or apple cider.

Gas production can often be traced to high roughage diets and to the consumption of "healthy" or "fancy" vegetables (broccoli, bean sprouts, asparagus, mushrooms, cabbage, etc). Raisins, dry fruits, and fruit rolls are popular snacks for toddlers and are consistent gas producers. Prunes, for example, contain a colonic stimulant. Overzealous attempts to control bowel movements can easily result in excessive flatus and cramps. Cereals high in bran will normally result in bulkier and more gas-containing stools. In fact, it is the gas trapped in the stool and not the fat content that accounts for its floatability. In some individuals gluten-containing products can result in excessive flatulence. This effect is totally different than the enteropathy caused by gliadin sensitivity.

A systematic dietary history and judicious step-wise manipulation of the intake will, in most cases, clarify the source of gas and simplify its management. The use of activated charcoal can provide some symptomatic relief but more effective long-term results are obtained by understanding and changing the diet.

# BIBLIOGRAPHY

1. Levitt MD: Production and excretion of hydrogen gas in man. *N Engl J Med* 1969; 281:122–127.
2. Levitt MD, Duane WC: Floating stools: Flatus versus fat. *N Engl J Med* 1972; 286:973–975.
3. Levitt MD, Bond JH: Flatulence. *Ann Rev Med* 1980; 31:127–137.
4. Hickey CA, Calloway DH, and Murphy EL: Intestinal gas production following ingestion of fruits and fruit juices. *Am J Dig Dis* 1972; 17:383–389.
5. Potter T, Ellis C, Levitt M: Activated charcoal: In vivo and in vitro studies of effect on gas formation. *Gastroenterology* 1985; 88:620–624.
6. Gauderer MWL, Halpin TC, Izant RJ: Pathologic childhood aerophagia: A recognizable clinical entity. *J Pediatr Surg* 1981; 16:301–305.

# 8

# Abdominal Pains

Pain arising from structures in the abdomen is a frequent complaint, either volunteered by the patient or inferred by the parents from gestures, associated vomiting, or changes in bowel movements. A systematic approach to the symptom is useful in screening for more serious and urgent problems since one of the most important considerations in the workup of a child with abdominal pains is sorting out whether the pain is due to an intra-abdominal process needing prompt surgical intervention, or whether it results from physiological disturbances which can be investigated out in a more leisurely way.

Parents often instinctively ascribe pains to abdominal sources unless other obvious reasons account for the discomfort. A severe diaper rash or crying in association with voiding will always be perceived as a less worrisome situation. When pain is more obscure in nature, anxiety levels are bound to escalate, often compounded by feelings of helplessness.

In the assessment and evaluation of abdominal pain, one depends heavily on the parents' impressions and their interpretation of the child's responses. Some parents have a low threshold for their own pain and will often become extremely anxious and project their own sympathy to the child. The task of the practitioner is to take into consideration all of these extraneous factors and read through them, paying attention to the message and filtering out unnecessary distractions (Table 8–1).

TABLE 8–1.
Key Questions to Answer in the Evaluation of
Abdominal Pain

Age
Duration
Mode of onset
Location and extension
Quality of the pain (continuous, crampy)
Intensity
Precipitating and mitigating factors: movement, immobility
Nocturnal occurrence
Associated symptoms: nausea, vomiting, anorexia
Concomitant changes: pallor, fever, jaundice

# MECHANISMS OF ABDOMINAL PAIN

It is useful to think of abdominal pain in physiological terms. A basic understanding of the mechanisms involved in pain production, transmission, and perception is crucial for a logical assessment and provides the necessary framework
to guide the questioning and to direct the investigation.

Pain in the abdominal cavity can be derived from:

1. The intestinal tract and its associated organs (liver, gallbladder, spleen,
pancreas).
2. Their peritoneal covering, both visceral and parietal.
3. Nongastrointestinal structures, kidneys, ureters, bladder, and spine.

Extra-abdominal organs can also refer pain to the abdomen as is the case
in some cases of pneumonia, pleuritis, or pericarditis.

# DEVELOPMENTAL AND PHYSIOLOGICAL ASPECTS

During the development of the organism, blood vessels and nerves appear seg-
mentally and progress to their intended targets through a process of migration
and rotation. This segmental distribution helps explain referred pain, and is often
a useful clue in discriminating somatic from visceral pain (Fig 8–1). The in-
dependence among autonomic and somatic innervation is functionally less clear
than previously considered. Consequently, reflexes triggered by somatic afferent
fibers can produce visceral responses, and, conversely, visceral stimuli can result
in somatic responses. Nerve impulses originating in visceral structures are transmitted through branches of the sympathetic nervous system and travel through
larger, myelinated fibers typically resulting in poorly localized sensations often

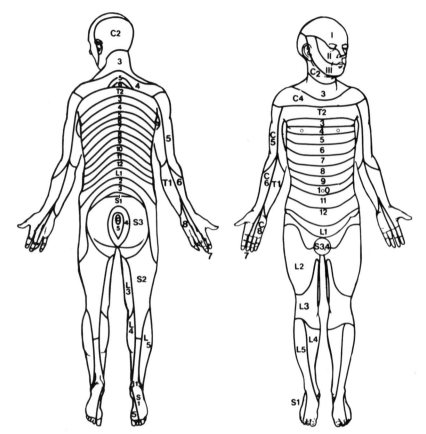

**FIG 8–1.**
Segmental nerve distribution. Recognition of the dermatomal areas innervated by
a specific spinal nerve is useful in understanding patterns of referred pain. (From
Currie DJ: *Abdominal Pain.* New York, Hemisphere Publishing Corp, 1979. Used
by permission.)

overlapping adjacent segments. In contrast, pain arising from nerve endings in
somatic sensory afferents is sharp, well defined, and almost pinpoint in quality.
These characteristics are of great importance in the clinical evaluation of the
patient with pain.

Pain in the intestinal tract is produced by three basic stimuli: (1) distention
or contraction of a hollow viscus, (2) ischemic compromise, and (3) some noxious
chemically mediated stimuli.

Pain in the solid viscera is derived from pain receptors in their capsules,
although sensation from the hepatic and pancreatic parenchyma can be traced to
branches of the sympathetic nervous system found in close apposition to veins
and arterioles.

The pathophysiologic explanation of the sequence of events taking place during an attack of appendicitis is useful in the understanding of these concepts. As presently understood, the initial event in acute appendicitis is an obstruction, partial or complete, of the appendiceal lumen. The pain is transmitted first through the visceral afferent nerves arising from spinal segments T9–T10, being perceived as diffuse periumbilical discomfort. Frequently associated with the obstruction, vagally mediated impulses produce nausea and vomiting. As the venous return from the appendix is compromised, the mesentery becomes edematous and stretches the serosa which has by now become inflamed. The parietal peritoneum, through somatic branches afferent to the T10 spinal level, will localize the pain to McBurney's point. If the appendix is in a retrocecal position, the point of irritation of the parietal peritoneum will be in the back or even in the right upper quadrant. If perforation occurs, the abdominal musculature responds with spasm, rigidity, and hyperesthesia.

### Clinical Evaluation

Very often, the physician will be consulted about the child's distress over the phone. If the onset of the abdominal pain is sudden, the first issue is whether the patient should be brought to the office or should be directed to an emergency room. To help with these determinations, an idea of the different diagnostic entities that affect children in various age groups is useful (Table 8–2). Certain

TABLE 8–2.
Conditions Responsible for Abdominal Pain
Medically Manageable

*Infants*
　Colic/fussiness
　Formula intolerance (carbohydrates, protein)
　Gastroenteritis (viral, bacterial, parasitic)
　Rectal fissure
　Aerophagia

*Older Children and Teenagers*
　Indigestion
　Constipation/fecal impaction
　Gastroenteritis (viral, bacterial, rickettsial, food poisoning)
　Mesenteric adenitis
　Pelvic inflammatory disease
　Hepatitis/pancreatitis
　Inflammatory bowel disease (ileitis/colitis)
　Bacterial peritonitis
　Midcycle (ovulatory) pains: "Mittleschmerz"
　Henoch-Schönlein purpura/lupus/rheumatic fever
　Sickle-cell crisis
　Ketoacidosis/uremia

*(continued)*

TABLE 8–2.  *Continued*

*Older Children and Teenagers*

Adrenal insufficiency
Lead poisoning
Polyserositis (familial Mediterranean fever)
Herpes zoster

*Extraintestinal Sources*
Lower lobe pneumonia
Hydronephrosis/pyelonephritis

complications such as swallowing difficulties associated with tracheoesophageal fistula and esophageal atresia, vomiting associated with intestinal obstruction secondary to atresia, or aganglionosis are present in early infancy. As the child gets older, and usually within the first 6 weeks of life, pyloric stenosis is more likely to occur in the child with protracted vomiting. Infectious and metabolic abnormalities need to also be considered in the child with vomiting. Symptomatic abdominal distention in a toddler is more likely to be due to intussusception or malrotation. A list of age-related diagnoses appears in Table 8–3.

An objective examiner will be able to bring together clinical acumen and inquisitive prodding in order to elicit as much information as possible prior to proceeding with laboratory investigations. A detailed medical history is the single most useful tool in the diagnosis of abdominal pain. If the child is old enough, it is important to ask for first-hand information; there is a lot to learn from the mouths of babes!

If one approaches the child with abdominal pains in a systematic fashion and attention is given to accompanying findings such as vomiting, jaundice, pallor, or distention, the problem can usually be sorted out without delay.

## COLIC

A certain amount of crying is part of the normal physiologic (and probably psychologic) development of the infant. Nothing generates more anxiety in parents than seeing their baby scream in apparent agony, with very little to offer and the belief that there must be a reason for the pain. It is difficult to convince the family who is faced with an infant who screams and thrashes for hours that nothing is seriously wrong and that there is a reasonable explanation for what they are experiencing.

Understanding colic or rather, the colicky temperament, is going to allow the pediatrician to offer guidance, reassurance, and reasonable expectations. Offering reassurances or dismissing the importance of the symptom at an early stage could develop into an embarrassing situation if the child happens to have been injured by an open safety pin (not too frequent in these days of disposable diapers), or has intussusception or peptic esophagitis.

Obviously, the first step in the effective management of colic is to rule out systemic disease with a thorough history and physical examination. It is not surprising that colic should be suspected of being gastrointestinal in origin. The infant's movements, feeding behavior, and unhappiness are easily attributed to gas, hunger, intestinal cramping, constipation, or formula intolerance.

## What Is Colic?

Colic is most likely a complex of general physiologic immaturity of the nervous system. This "imbalance" also affects the gastrointestinal tract, so rich in in-

TABLE 8–3.
Common Sources of Abdominal Pain Usually Resulting in Surgical Intervention

*Infants*
  Acute distention
  Pyloric stenosis
  Intestinal obstruction
  Malrotation/volvulus
  Aganglionosis
  Imperforated anus
  Incarcerated hernia (epigastric, umbilical, inguinal, femoral, obturator)
  Testicular or ovarian torsion
  Renal cysts
  Perforated viscus
    Gastric/duodenal ulcer
    Enterocolitis
    Appendicitis

*Older Children and Teenagers*
  Intussusception
  Meckel's diverticulum
  Malrotation/volvulus
  Incarcerated hernia
  Appendicitis
  Peptic ulcers
  Esophagitis
  Gallbladder/bile duct inflammation/stones
  Traumatic injury to duodenum/liver
  Spine tumor with nerve compression
  Obstruction renal calculi
  Testicular torsion/ovarian cyst hemorrhage
  Ectopic pregnancy

nervation and constantly stimulated by feedings and peristalsis. The choice of the term *colic* is partly responsible for the common perception as an intestinal entity (from the Greek *kolon*, meaning large intestine). Interpreting colic as a simple exaggerated response of the intestine to distention is not very useful. Mechanistic approaches with measures primarily aimed at relieving gas (frequent burping, suppositories, thermometers, etc.), sedating the child or trying every imaginable formula, will usually result in more bewilderment and endless frustration both for the physician and the parents.

Frantic phone calls in the middle of the night can be minimized if the parents have some insight into the symptom complex and understand that serious illness has been ruled out and that the condition is self-limited. It is far better to try simple measures and give support and reassurance rather than experimenting with new methods of crying control.

## Patterns of Crying

The pattern of crying in colic is not always typical. The onset tends to be sudden, a crying attack beginning out of the blue, usually in the evening (accumulated nervous tension needing venting?). It can last for hours and sometimes cease only when the infant is exhausted. Exhaustion by itself can cause frantic crying. Crying is accompanied by fussiness, agitation, inconsolable screaming, and body stiffness. The face turns purple, the eyes and fists are clenched shut, and the picture is one of agonizing suffering and misery. Yet, for all we know, stress without physical pain can produce identical behavior. This can be used as a reassuring argument for the parents. For a few minutes the infant stops, usually when being fed. Gulping is common. Feedings are given on demand trying to bring some silence into the household. More often than not, feedings do not seem to satisfy the baby for long. On the contrary, they seem to be the most immediate cause of persistent crying. Anxiety rises by the hour, and sleepless nights contribute to the parents' frustration. Tension among the parents is usually further compounded by a bombardment of free advice offered by well meaning friends and relatives. Normal babies also cry 2–3 hours a day during the first 6 weeks of life, and colic probably represents an excessive crying above those "norms."

### Etiologies of Colic
Unfortunately, a definite explanation for this symptom complex is still missing. Some of the most popular theories proposed over the years have included:

1. Aerophagia/faulty feeding methods.
2. Hormonal/neurological (hypertonicity).
3. Food allergies/intolerances (lactose, caffeine, iron).
4. Environmental.

5. Tense parent-child interaction/inappropriate handling.

Because it is so difficult to prove a food allergy, this theory has been repeatedly explored with elimination diets and the use of hypoallergenic formulas. The beneficial effect of changing a formula that contains cow's protein to one based on soy or hydrolyzed casein is often difficult to confirm. Frequently, every new change seems to help a little for a brief time, only to return to the starting point just when things appeared to be finally getting under control. Most recently, consumption of milk products by the lactating mother has been advanced as a treatable reason for colic in close to one third of breast-fed babies with this symptom. Unfortunately, serious methodological questions hamper the acceptance of those conclusions. Other studies suggest that breast-fed babies are more prone to colic, postulating a colic-producing factor in the milk. Lactose intolerance is not a common reason for colic. The effect of low progesterone levels on colic was proposed in the past, but these results have not been confirmed.

Strained parent-child interaction, whether primary or secondary, is almost always part of the picture. Insecurity on the part of the mother or father, feelings of helplessness, and depression often contribute to the tense atmosphere in the household. Disharmony, mutual criticism, frustration, and sheer exhaustion build up high emotional levels. The ways in which an infant perceives this tension and reacts to it are not well understood. Changes in the way a baby is held, rocked, fed, talked to, or looked at must trigger overreactivity. Often, the severity of the colic seems to diminish when the child is consistently handled without panic, anger, or guilt feelings.

### Management Pointers

Understanding that crying by itself is not a reason to pick up the baby immediately and that sometimes the baby will quiet down faster if left alone will help modify the instinctive reactions of anxious parents. Frequent dialogue with the parents, support, and positive reinforcement can sometimes considerably modify the course of colic.

Recommending a couple of ounces of water or sugar water after a long spell of crying might help relieve gastric air and decrease intestinal cramping associated with aerophagia. Finding someone to watch over the baby for a few hours does a great deal of good and should be encouraged. Above all, the parents should feel that the hysterical crying is not a proof of their incompetence, but rather a developmental phase and an expression of their child's temperament and interaction with the environment. Certain maneuvers can be tried and, surprisingly, seem to work at times. If nothing else, it gives the parents something concrete to do while the days and the nights go by.

The use of medications alone is not as effective as intervention that combines psychological and behavioral modifications. Some parents are reluctant to use psychotropic medications in their infants and should not be forced into it. Preparations containing anticholinergic agents such as homatropine, methyl bromide, or belladonna alkaloids (hyoscyamine, scopolamine), phenobarbital, antiflatulents (simethicone), or antihistamines (diphenhydramine) are frequently tried in an attempt to calm the baby. One should always be cautious while using these medications in young infants. Paradoxical reactions, ileus, overdose, tachyphylaxis, and even withdrawal symptoms can complicate an essentially benign and self-limited condition.

*Prognosis*
    The practitioner can in most cases affect the course of colic if support and guidance are coupled with thoroughness in the search for a treatable cause of excessive crying. A more encompassing philosophy about the origins and dynamics of this condition, and attention to the parent-infant interaction, will prove more useful than stop-gap measures and trial and error intervention.

## RECURRENT ABDOMINAL PAIN

The child presenting with a history of recurrent or persistent abdominal pains will often challenge the diagnostic skills and patience of even the most seasoned doctor. Appropriately, Levine paraphrased the experience as the "loneliness of the long distance physician" in his excellent conceptual monograph on the subject.
    The gastrointestinal tract is one of the organs most vulnerable to somatization, not surprising considering the complex interactions between the autonomic nervous system, with its rich innervation to the gut, and the influence of higher cortical centers. Frequently, complaints will also include headaches or pain in the extremities. Autonomic instability has been suggested by the associated pallor, flushing, and sweatiness accompanying the pain attacks. Other studies have demonstrated enhanced pupillary reactions and vasomotor hyperreactivity in some children with this syndrome.

### Definition and Epidemiology

John Apley in his classic study of the syndrome in 1,000 British school children defined recurrent abdominal pain as pain occurring three or more times in the 3 months preceding presentation and resulting in disruption of normal activities. He found girls were affected slightly more than boys (12% vs. 10%) and onset increased from age 5 years until age 7. Between the ages of 5 to 10 years, 10.8% of the population he followed fulfilled his diagnostic criteria. Other surveys have confirmed these incidence rates in other Western populations, with exceptionally high figures in some studies involving adolescents (up to 30%). Although it is reassuring to think that 90% of children investigated for recurrent abdominal pains will be free of organic disease, the first priority in the assessment of a new patient is to be able to identify from the outset the other 10%. Nothing is more embarrassing than to spend several visits discussing the psychosocial dimensions of recurrent pain, only to find out that Familial Mediterranean Fever, intermittent hydronephrosis, Crohn's disease, or a spinal tumor were responsible for the symptoms all along. Even more distressing is when the right diagnosis is made by someone else (second or third opinions!).

Special attention is necessary when dealing with certain childhood populations where gastrointestinal parasites and infections are unusually high. In these children, organic and easily treatable abdominal pain can account for more than 60% of the cases.

### Evaluation

The only protection against this diagnostic pitfall is a thorough and open-minded evaluation of the patient from the very first visit. Enough time should be allocated for the initial consult, and many hours and phone calls can be saved by the comprehensive and objective physician who takes the trouble to take a good history, systems review, and psychosocial profile. Often, sensitive information will not be volunteered in the first encounter, but encouragement and a positive, nonjudgmental attitude can help open communication. Considering the chronicity of the symptoms in many of the patients, the doctor should strive to offer reassurance, suggesting sensitive areas in the life of the child that need to be looked into, and provide sensible advice. None of this can be done when an antagonistic relationship has been allowed to develop between the doctor and the patient's family. It is difficult to feel helpful when all recommendations fail to improve the symptoms and parental frustration and anxiety turns into skepticism and silent (or verbal) questioning of the doctor's abilities.

### Clinical Features

Severe abdominal pain of acute onset can be the initial presentation of the syndrome, and only the subsequent clinical course will allow proper identification and classification. Unfortunately, there are no particular features that will make the diagnosis of nonorganic pain fail-safe. In general, pain tends to be periumbilical and vaguely localized. The more localized the pain is, the greater the likelihood of organic disease, especially if the localization is epigastric, right upper quadrant (with radiation to the shoulder or flank), and right lower quadrant. Very localized pain is suggestive of a musculoskeletal origin, frequently under the costal margin or along the recti.

Attacks can either be brief, lasting a few minutes, or most frequently, pain can linger on for hours, during which time the child lies down or appears in various degrees of discomfort. Nothing seems to help. The child looks pale and tired, and sometimes drowsy and dizzy after the episode. Nausea, vomiting, leg pains, headaches, loose stools or constipation can also be associated with the attacks, but no distinctive pattern is usually present. More importantly, none of these symptoms can help distinguish between pain of organic or nonorganic origin, so that an objective examination is needed in every case, several times if necessary.

A family history of functional and psychogenic disorders is not unusual (up to 50% in some series), involving the gastrointestinal tract, ill-defined allergies, or the central nervous system (headaches, migraines, tension). In some patients, a history of difficulties during the pregnancy or delivery can be obtained, and up to 25% of children have a history of colic as infants.

## Psychological Aspects

A most important area to explore in the evaluation of the child with recurrent pain is the presence of stress in the household and in the school. Often there are marital strains or the recent loss of a loved one (including family pets). School problems can be overt or very subtle. Academic excellence is a source of satisfaction to the highly motivated student and his family, but success sometimes comes at the expense of continuous pressure to maintain the high standards of achievement, and social interactions with peers can suffer in the process. Being singled out by a demanding or picky teacher or feeling isolated or harassed by students can force a child to escape the unfriendly school atmosphere by having a symptom beyond his or her control. School absenteeism can become a problem by itself if allowed to continue while the child complains of pain. The early morning pain attack usually results in the child missing school. If the child is pressured to go to school, a phone call from the nurse or the principal might force the parents to come and pick the child up, a difficult situation if, as is often the case, both parents work. School-related stress needs to be explored with teachers, counselors, and friends. Arrangements to help the child make up for lost exams and prevent further lags while the situation is being resolved can be very useful, as long as it is temporary and not a crutch or an easy way out.

## Physical Examination

The child may appear quite healthy during the exam, and will often be less concerned about the medical problems than the accompanying parent. An effort should be made to let the child speak for him- or herself, avoiding constant cueing or visual approval from the parent. Positioning the patient closer to the desk as the parent sits behind can provide a natural separation and afford a more direct line of communication between the doctor and the child.

Signs of organic disease to look for include:

• Jaundice
• Conjunctival pallor
• Muscle wasting

- Weight/height disproportion
- Fever
- Mucosal lesions
- Dermatomal distribution of pain or rash
- Chronic cough
- Abdominal distention and organomegaly
- Prominent venous pattern
- Abdominal mass
- Perianal lesions
- Occult blood in stool or urine.

Frequent findings in the typical recurrent abdominal pain syndrome include diffuse tenderness to deep palpation, stool in the sigmoid or transverse colon, and hard stool in the ampulla on rectal examination. Although the causal relation between constipation and pellet-like stools and the etiology of the syndrome remains unproven, it is not difficult to blame the presence of hard stool for painful colonic spasms. This also can give a "way out" to the child once advice and a simple regimen of stool lubrication or fiber is prescribed. It is likely that a motility dysfunction is one of the important factors underlying the pathophysiology of the syndrome.

### Laboratory and Other Investigations

Basic laboratory tests will help rule out organic disease and should be performed at the initial evaluation. Negative results will lend more weight to one's reassurances and conservative approach.

Initial tests include:

- Complete blood count and differential
- Sedimentation rate
- Urine analysis
- Sequential Multiple Analysis (SMA-12 or similar: liver functions, creatinine, BUN, etc.)
- Amylase
- Stool guaiac
- Abdominal scout film (vertebral abnormalities, fecalith, stool impaction).

An abdominal ultrasonogram can be useful in ruling out cholelithiasis, obstructive kidney disease, ovarian pathology, and in the detection of abnormal masses.

Depending on these results and on the clinical course, the need for more studies can be determined:

- Breath hydrogen for carbohydrate malabsorption
- Upper GI and small bowel follow through

• Abdominal computerized axial tomograph
• Intravenous pyelogram
• Barium enema
• Upper and lower endoscopy
• Pelvic examination.

Lactose intolerance often presents with crampy pains, nausea, diarrhea, and bloatedness, but studies in populations of children with the syndrome of recurrent abdominal pains have failed to document that this is a significant factor in its etiology in most patients. Obviously, an accurate history will suggest the diagnosis of disaccharidase deficiency and will permit effective management.

## Management

An important aspect in the management of nonorganic abdominal pains is to avoid the pitfall of assuming that "there must be something wrong" with the patient to account for the persistent symptoms. Once the possibility of serious organic disease has been reasonably ruled out, the continued search for a structural explanation for the pain with more aggressive investigations (including exploratory laparotomy or laparoscopy) should be discouraged. This usually conveys the impression that the doctor is not convinced of his or her evaluation, and it only helps reinforce the hypochondriacal fears of the patient and the family.

Counseling and supportive guidance is the treatment of choice in children with recurrent pains and their families. Developing a good rapport and being able to discuss important aspects of the psychodynamics of the family are more helpful than any drug therapy. The use of antispasmodics, antidepressants, anticonvulsants, or narcotics adds the risk of potentially troublesome side effects and has not been proven more effective than placebo in controlled trials.

The practitioner or the consultant gastroenterologist is usually in a good position to offer advice and serve as a sounding board for problems in the household or in the school. Reassurance that no organic disturbance is present needs to be offered time and time again to anxious parents, while one tries to reduce tensions and attempt modification of certain behavior patterns, especially the parents' reactions to their child's complaints. If more serious psychological derangements are detected or chaotic family interactions are present, a referral to a psychiatric social worker, psychologist, or psychiatrist is indicated.

## Prognosis

More than one-third of children presenting with the syndrome of recurrent abdominal pains will continue to experience psychosomatic complaints as they grow into adulthood. In some, the symptoms will involve other vulnerable areas (headaches, gynecological complaints, irritable bowel). In most series with long-term follow-up (3 to 30 years), the diagnosis of missed organic disease was made in only a small minority of patients.

## BIBLIOGRAPHY

1. Silen W: *Cope's Early Diagnosis of the Acute Abdomen*, ed 15. New York, Oxford University Press, 1979.
2. Currie DJ: *Abdominal Pain*. New York, Hemisphere Publishing Corporation, 1979.
3. Wessel MA, Cobb JC, Jackson EB et al: Paroxysmal fussing in infancy, sometimes called colic. *Pediatrics* 1954; 14:421–435.
4. Carey WB: ''Colic'' — primary excessive crying as an infant — environment interaction. *Pediatr Clin North Am* 1984; 31(5):993–1005.
5. Brazelton TB: Crying in infancy. *Pediatrics* 1962; 29:579–588.
6. Apley J: *The Child with Abdominal Pains*, ed 2. Boston, Blackwell Scientific Publications, 1975.
7. Levine MD, Rappaport LA: Recurrent abdominal pain in school children: The loneliness of the long-distance physician. *Pediatr Clin North Am* 1984; 31(5) 969–991.
8. Davidson M: Recurrent abdominal pain: Look to dyskinesia as the culprit. *Contemp Pediatr* 1986; 3:16–42.

# 9

# Constipation

Constipation refers to infrequent passage of stools, increased hardness or size of the movements, or difficulties with the process of passing a stool. It is important to obtain a clear description of what the parent means when the term is used, since in many instances, perfectly normal patterns of defecation are being misinterpreted due to personal, familial, or social expectations. On the other hand, some parents are perfectly happy with one or two movements every day or every other day, without realizing that this infrequency could be of significance when compared to other children of the same age.

## EXPECTED STOOLING PATTERNS

Premature infants will frequently display colonic atony. Maturational factors play a role in the establishment of normal propulsive contractions; as the infant grows, coordination and effectiveness of the mass peristalsis improves. In the full-term infant, the gastrocolic reflex is usually present at birth and a bowel movement during or shortly after a feeding is commonplace. The breast-fed infant has on average 5 to 7 stools a day. This number decreases to 1 to 3 per day during the second half of the first year of life.

# FUNCTIONAL ANATOMY OF DEFECATION

## SENSORY                              MOTOR

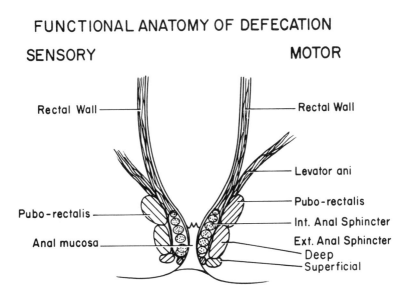

**FIG 9–1.**
Main anatomical mechanisms responsible for fecal continence. (From Welch KJ, Randolph JG, Ravitch MM, et al: *Pediatric Surgery*, ed 4. Chicago, Year Book Medical Publishers, 1986. Used by permission.)

When the newborn has many less movements than expected (only one or two per day), the possibility of a predisposition for constipation should be considered. Close attention to the progression of the stooling patterns and to the difficulties associated with passage of the bowel movements can help modify, and in many cases effectively control, the development of later age stool withholding and more deep-rooted constipation.

## MECHANISMS OF CONTINENCE

The development of fecal continence is dependent on a number of structural and functional factors. Voluntary control is established during the process of toilet training; this depends on proper central nervous system function. Mental retardation can result in incontinence even if all the neuronal pathways are intact. Social customs will determine to a certain extent the age of toilet training and the stress placed on the parents and child when those attempts are not successful at the expected time.

The major components of the apparatus of defecation are sensory and motor elements (Fig 9–1).

## Sensory Elements

Perceptions from the rectal ampulla arise from stretch receptors in its wall, and travel through the spinal cord to complete the sacroanal reflex. Sensory afferents in the muscles of the pelvic floor probably also contribute to the sensation of rectal fullness. Defects in sensory innervation at this level and abnormal rectal sensation can seriously impair continence. Less important is the perception of anal canal sensations.

Up to a certain threshold, central inhibitory control is possible when the ampulla is distended. Above that limit, involuntary motor contractions and emptying occur. Interconnections with the higher centers affecting voluntary control take place at the level of S1–4.

Below the pectinate line in the anal canal, distinctions can be made between pain, temperature, and pressure, but not as precise as the sensations emanating from the perianal skin. These sensations are mediated via superficial pudendal afferents. Above the pectinate line, only distention is perceived.

## Motor Elements

The three major muscle groups involved in continence are the internal anal sphincter, the levator ani with its puborectalis sling, and the external anal sphincter. They all play important roles and are structurally interesting, being striated muscles under autonomic nervous system modulation (levator ani and external anal sphincter) and smooth muscle with continuous contractile activity (internal sphincter) responsible for maintaining its resting pressure.

The levator ani and its branch, the puborectalis sling, are of outmost importance in maintaining the angulation between the axis of the alimentary canal above and the anal canal below. A group of muscles from the puborectalis splits in two and envelopes the area of the internal sphincter attaching anteriorly to the pubis. When in a state of contraction, which is under voluntary control via the internal pudendal nerves, the sling maintains an angle of about 80 degrees between the two canals. Weakness of the puborectalis can be checked during the rectal examination by pulling the rectum toward the coccyx. The anal canal will open widely when weakness is present. Neurological lesions, repeated rectal prolapse, or injury to the puborectalis or sphincters will result in incontinence.

When the fecal mass reaches the puborectalis, one can either relax this muscle group and allow the stool to enter the anal canal, or, by causing it to contract, increase the angulation and prevent passage of stool into the ampulla.

## CAUSES OF CHILDHOOD CONSTIPATION

The two most common mechanisms for constipation in the child are difficulty with expulsion of the stool and drying of the fecal mass in the colon, usually a result of muscle spasm and close opposition between the mucosa and the stool. As the muscle tone increases in the rectum and colon, water reabsorption seems to increase or becomes more effective, contributing to the formation of the familiar scybala.

*Delayed gastric emptying* of food and abnormally slow transit times can sometimes be the underlying cause of constipation, and children with pyloric stenosis or other congenital defects (malrotation, Ladd's bands) can have constipation. *Motility disorders* affecting part of or the whole gastrointestinal tract are being discovered with recent developments in investigative techniques. Isotope-labelled food is used to calculate gastric emptying time, and the use of markers has allowed monitoring of intestinal transit times. In some cases of constipation due to abnormal physiological mechanisms (transit or colonic tone and motility), constitutional factors are at play, and studies in identical twins confirm the genetic nature of the predisposition for constipation.

*Metabolic disorders* can have a more or less prominent effect on intestinal function, and constipation is encountered in states resulting in hypokalemia, hypothyroidism, hyperparathyroidism, or lead poisoning. It is always important to rule out these conditions (on clinical and, if necessary, laboratory grounds) whenever approaching the child with constipation. In addition, commonly used medications such as aluminum- or calcium-containing antacids, cough syrups with codeine, other opiates, and anticholinergics can result in distressing constipation from delayed transit or increased water reabsorption in the distal colon.

Commonly, constipation results from *voluntary withholding* and other difficulties at the time of the bowel movements. Conditioned reflexes can create a pattern of pain or discomfort-avoidance if the process is accompanied by pain or if anal fissures or other lesions complicate the picture.

Although the role of the abdominal muscles in normal defecation is not crucial, children with weak abdominal musculature (neuromuscular disease, agenesis of the abdominal muscles, etc.) can suffer from constipation. If the innervation to the anorectal segments is affected by demyelinating diseases, spinal cord injury, or a sacral tumor, constipation (and sometimes, urinary retention as well) can be a major problem. An inquiry about urinary function is an important part of the evaluation of the child with constipation or incontinence.

Imperforate anus should be looked for in every newborn, and is, of course, a reason for absolute constipation. More difficult to diagnose are other *abnormalities of rectal placement* and stricturing, which nonetheless should be detectable by careful physical examination and rectal examination. Stimulation of the anal area with a Q-tip can show the location of a displaced sphincter or help demonstrate a rectal shelf. The incidence of stenosis responsible for mechanical interference with passage of stool is very small, and the practice of anal dilatations should be discouraged. In most full-term infants, the anus accommodates the small finger during a digital examination. Pain and spasm are normal responses to such examinations and should not be interpreted as a sign of an abnormally narrowed canal.

## STOOL WITHHOLDING

As previously mentioned, stool retention is probably one of the most common reasons for constipation in the toddler and older child. If the retention is long-lasting, mechanical stretching of the rectum and sigmoid can result in a markedly dilated structure ("megarectum") which is able to accommodate large volumes of fecal material without sending urgent messages to the cortex. Initially, as the child finds it difficult and painful to empty the rectum, all sorts of maneuvers are attempted to keep the stool from dilating the rectal canal. Keeping the buttocks tightly closed, holding on to chairs or stairs, "duty dancing," or sitting on the floor in a semireclining position all accomplish the goal of forcing the stool mass back into the sigmoid.

The role of the puborectalis sling in straightening the angulation between the rectum and the anal canal is important in promoting efficient emptying. This sling becomes tighter when the distance between the spine and the pubis are greatest, and this is the case when the child is in a fully seated or squatting position, with the legs firmly pressing on the floor. Conversely, when the sling is relaxed, as occurs during standing or in the semirecumbent position, the angulation between the anal canal and the rectum is maximal, and attempts to expel the stool will be ineffectual no matter how much abdominal wall contraction and Valsalva maneuvering are exerted. During the process, the child turns beet red, sweats, seems in agony, and does not want to be approached or handled. This is a clear sign that the apparatus of defecation is intact, and that the child is able to sense the stool movement into the rectum. Once the stool is pushed back, the urgency subsides and the child will be relieved, at least temporarily. It is not unusual to hear descriptions of a pale, lethargic, or whiny child at the end of the episode.

In a way, the expression of difficulties moving the bowels so frequently heard from parents is a reassurance that constipation is due to stool withholding and not to abnormal innervation or abnormal muscular development of the intestine, the parents' most common fear. In contrast, in Hirschsprung's disease, the spastic segment prevents the descent of the stool bulk, and therefore there is no sensation of urgency.

### Management of Constipation

In the infant with sparse movement and associated straining, the easiest approach includes the use of lubricated Q-tip or glycerin suppository. If a thermometer is used, care should be taken in proper instructions to prevent slippage or breakage. A change of formula can also be tried, since some children tend to have looser movements when receiving a soy-based milk. At times, constipation is reported in some children receiving soy formulas, and a change to a different preparation or to a lactose-containing milk might bring good results.

After age 3–4 months, it is possible to modify transit time and stool bulk with a fiber supplement such as Maltsupex which contains indigestible malt and fermenting dextrins (carbohydrate). Corn syrup is prescribed for the same reason, but does not have the advantage of containing a bulking agent, and if used in excess, can considerably increase the caloric intake and result in overweight. In the older child, mineral oil can safely be used to prevent excessive drying of the stool and promote painless emptying. Lactulose can be used for the same purpose. Later, if difficulties persist, a mild colonic stimulant containing senna or cascara can be tried. The goal is to prevent the establishment of a pattern of delayed rectal emptying and progressive obstipation since a protracted course will be likely to result in encopresis from seepage of unformed stool around an impaction.

## BIBLIOGRAPHY

1. Clayden GS, Lawson J: Investigation and management of long standing chronic constipation in children. *Arch Dis Child* 1976; 51:918–923.
2. Davidson M, Kugler MM, Baver CH: Diagnosis and management in children with severe and protracted constipation and obstipation. *J. Pediatr* 1963; 62:261–275.
3. Bentley JFR: Constipation in infants and children: Progress report. *Gut* 1971; 12:85–90.
4. Shoffner CE: Urinary tract pathology associated with constipation. *Radiology* 1978; 90:865–877.
5. Safety of stool softeners. *Med Lett Drugs Ther* 1977; 19(11):45.
6. Duthie HL: Defecation and the anal sphincters. *Clin Gastroenterol* 1982; 11(3):621–631.
7. Fritz GK, Armbrust J: Eneuresis and encopresis. *Psychiatr Clin North Am* 1982; 5(2):283–295.
8. Abrahamian FP, Lloyd-Still JD: Chronic constipation in childhood: Longitudinal study of 186 patients. *J Pediatr Gastroenterol Nutr* 1984; 3:460–467.

# Encopresis

Encopresis is a term used to describe the soiling of underpants and clothes with stool, whether this occurs consciously or involuntarily. Although usually associated with constipation, it is not synonymous with it. However, encopresis without underlying fecal impaction (the so-called "nonretentive soiling") is seen in a small minority of patients. It can be a symptom of a serious behavioral and psychiatric disorder. Management of the disorder can be one of the most frustrating aspects of common pediatric care.

The problem is seen in all socioeconomic groups and is more common in boys than in girls (4–5:1). Its incidence is highest in the 5- to 10-year-old age groups and diminishes with approaching adolescence. Occurrence in adolescents and adults is frequently associated with psychiatric disorders or mental retardation. In some situations, a family history of encopresis in one of the parents (usually the father) is also elicited.

It is important to be sure that the soiling is not secondary to *abnormal innervation* of the rectum with inability to maintain normal sphincter function or due to a progressive loss of function from a spinal cord tumor or a *tethered cord*. In those cases, a thorough neurological examination will detect other signs of spinal nerve involvement, often accompanied by bladder dysfunction as well.

# HISTORY

The history should elicit information on bowel and bladder function from the neonatal period, starting with the time of passage of meconium, frequency and consistency of bowel movements, and pattern of toilet training. Difficulties with motor milestones, hypotonia, recurrent urinary tract infections, and serious bouts of diarrhea can point to structural lesions.

On the other hand, if a history of chronic constipation or stool withholding is elicited and the child's development is otherwise normal, organic disorder is less likely. In most cases, it will not be possible to gather all the pertinent psychosocial information in a single session. It is important to take the necessary time to perform a thorough physical examination in the first visit, so that subsequent visits can concentrate on issues of retraining and family dynamics.

# RECTAL EXAMINATION

The rectal examination is obviously very useful. It gives an immediate indication of sensation and tone of the anal sphincter, the size of the ampulla, the presence of suspicious masses in the presacral area and associated lesions in the anal verge which can be responsible for painful stimuli at the time of defecation. It is also useful in helping determine whether more bowel cleaning is necessary or during treatment, especially when a recurrent impaction is suspected.

The importance of the rectal examination does not need to be emphasized. Anyone treating a child with encopresis must include it as part of the routine examination. Positive reinforcement can be given after an examination if improvement is noted. Some children will violently resist rectal examinations, in which case after the initial one, further correlations need to be done by abdominal palpation.

The management of the child with encopresis is within the realm of the pediatrician or primary physician, as long as treatment is approached in a consistent and physiologically oriented way. Additional consultations are sought when no progress is accomplished. Management is not easy or swift in most cases. On the contrary, it can be very time consuming and frustrating. The physician must be prepared to explore school and other social interactions, and often becomes the child's advocate.

## Etiology of Encopresis

Some controversy exists as to the origins and persistence of encopresis. Proponents of a primary colorectal dysfunction as the source of constipation, obstipation, fecal impaction, and stool seepage tend to be pragmatic in their treatment and report good success with this approach. This school concentrates on maintaining the colon empty of stools, reeducating the patient and the family in toilet training, and focusing less — at least initially — on the psychological and social implications of the symptom. Such an approach is cost effective and provides results faster than other techniques based on family psychotherapy and more intensive psychiatric intervention.

It is common and reassuring to find out that improved function and more normal attitudes surface when the symptom is improved, without the need for involved psychological intervention.

For this reason, it is recommended that, unless there are obvious deviations from normal in the parental relation to the child or in the psychological function of the child, a period of management concentrating on bowel habits and cleanup should precede family or individual therapy. It will be effective in many cases, and there is always time to bring the psychiatrist or psychologist into the picture if these initial maneuvers fail.

On the other hand, approaching the problem as a purely mechanical one is bound to fall short of expectations, and often ends up in impatience and frustration.

### Constitutional Factors

Recent manometric and electrophysiological investigations have revealed interesting findings supportive of the hypothesis that in some cases of functional constipation, deviations from normal are detectable in the threshold for relaxation of the internal sphincter, in the tone of the puborectalis muscle sling, and in colonic and rectal mass propulsive movements. Various combinations of those variations from normal are encountered in individual patients, and in some cases, in their families and twin siblings, suggesting a genetic predisposition to this kind of dysfunction.

In addition, the commonly expressed lack of urgency to defecate and the decreased perception of the presence of stool in the ampulla also have a physiological explanation, at least in part. Experimental studies in subjects with longstanding stool withholding confirm the decreased responsiveness to what would appear to be a major source of discomfort. With improvement in the muscle tone of the rectum and colon, perception threshold becomes more normal and can be a guide to the progress of medical management.

### Management of Encopresis

The four basic principles of the management of the child with encopresis are:

- Disimpaction of the rectum and colon
- Maintenance of a clean colon
- Establishment of more effective toilet habits
- Improvement in family and social interactions.

*Disimpaction*

Only in a minority of cases will the presenting impaction be severe enough to require hospitalization. In that case, high saline enemas are helpful. If the stool is too hard and wide, examination under anesthesia may be indicated to break the fecaloma manually and to mobilize the impaction. Some degree of mucosal friability can be present in protracted obstipation, and bleeding can occur at the time of the rectal examination. Spontaneous or induced "stercoral ulcers" can develop in rare instances, with considerable bleeding.

In the majority of cases, it will be possible to start the cleanup with a series of hypertonic phosphate enemas. Prepacked pediatric and adult sizes are convenient and safe, although there have been incidental reports of hyperphosphatemia and hypocalcemic tetanus following absorption of phosphate from the rectum. Better returns are obtained if the two enemas are given 1 hour apart. The following day, another phosphate or saline enema is given accompanied by a second one according to the results. Enemas are best administered with the child in the left-side-down position, and care should be taken not to introduce the tip of the enema directly into the mass of the stool, but rather to slide it alongside as far as possible. No pain should be felt if the enema is delivered slowly over 1–2 minutes. Sudden pain suggests expansion of the stool by an improperly positioned tip.

If necessary, enemas are given daily for 3 or 4 more days.

*Maintenance*

At the same time that colonic cleanup is in progress, the patient should be started on a maintenance regimen. One of the more commonly used ones was popularized by Davidson and coworkers in the 1960s, and is based on the use of large doses of mineral oil, sufficient to prevent reimpaction and to minimize the possibility of painful obstipation. Stool withholding also becomes more difficult as the stool is soft and lubricated.

An initial dosage can be in the range of an ounce for every 10 kg body weight, and it can all be given at once, nightly. Children usually object to the "sticky" texture of the oil on the tongue, but this can be minimized if offered in fruit juice or other tart drink. Some prefer it chilled or hidden in a milk shake or malted.

Parents frequently voice concern about the possibility of interference with vitamin absorption, but this has not been established and should even be less of a problem if the oil is given at nighttime, away from the food. If still unconvinced, a multivitamin supplement can be prescribed.

Mineral oil is continued for several months and the dosage adjusted according to the results. It is always important to confirm with a physical examination that stool accumulation is not occurring, before decreasing the dosage of oil because of leakage. A small amount of oil leakage is acceptable and sociably more tolerable than soiling and can be used as a guide in the tapering of the initial oil dosage. The maintenance dosage should be the minimal amount of oil which prevents recurrence of constipation and causes no oil leakage.

## Diet

For certain families, a wholesome diet with high roughage foodstuffs is commonplace and easy to maintain. In that environment, it is easy for children to get exposed to high-fiber diets and benefit from the improved colonic motility resulting when soft and bulky stools are present in the lumen. The situation is a little more complicated when a change is recommended in patients with less interest in fiber. It is worth explaining the advantages of this wholesome diet and offering some practical approaches to increasing the fiber content of everyday menus. Patient resistance to this kind of diet can be monumental. Energy should be spent in developing warm and caring relations with the child rather than with a stubborn fight over meals.

Fortunately, there are ways of increasing fiber intake with several preparations available in the market. Trial and error help determine the optimal dosage. It is useful to gain experience with a couple of formulations and become familiar with the best starting dosages and their expected effects. Most preparations are extracts of hydrophilic plants (psyllium, carrageenin) which absorb water and swell, becoming nonabsorbable bulk. High-fiber diets will normally produce more gas because of the effect of bacterial hydrolysis on the complex carbohydrates that constitute fiber. Patients should be advanced progressively to a higher residue diet, otherwise bloating and embarrassing flatus can occur. Another preparation (Kondremul) is an emulsion of mineral oil and fiber, which has been found to be useful in younger children since it is easily given by the spoon, dissolves in milk, and is mildly flavored.

## Establishment of Toilet Habits

While stool withholding is being minimized by keeping the stool soft and lubricated, the child should be encouraged to sit on the toilet at least twice a day. Parents should make sure that the feet are not dangling and can provide a small box or stool to give better leverage to the legs. It is not useful to spend more than 15 minutes at one sitting, and some authors have encouraged reading to shift the focus of attention.

Timing can be planned to take advantage of the gastrocolic reflex, a series of propulsive mass peristaltic movements triggered by ingestion of food. Convenient times are in the morning after breakfast and in the evening after dinner. For some children who tend to soil more after returning from school, the schedule can be modified accordingly.

Parents should not be trapped in a ritual of bathroom theatrics. They should maintain a neutrality, even when the visit has been successful. It is often found that the child will report not having to move his bowels at the time of his prescribed visit to the toilet. For that reason, the use of a senna laxative for 1 or 2 weeks can be helpful in increasing the urge to empty. The laxative should be given before bedtime so that its effect coincides with the morning movement. Alternative stimulation can be provided with a stimulant suppository (i.e., Dulcolax) in the morning.

In overweight children or when abdominal muscle tone is lax, exercise should be encouraged. It is not clear to what extent external compression of the colon contributes to evacuation, but attention to factors having a positive effect on the process of bowel emptying can help set up the right attitude and ultimately contribute to improved function.

## Impaired Family Relationships

Attempts to treat encopresis on a purely mechanical level will frequently become a constant source of frustration to the family and the physician alike. Only in the more simple cases of sudden onset obstipation with overflow incontinence will the maintenance of a clean colon effect an immediate cure. In the majority of cases, by the time the problem has been brought to the surface, psychological and social disruption has already occurred, at times very seriously. Undoing the damage to the patient's self-image and dealing with parental anger and ambivalence is not an easy task and requires time and patience.

In certain cases, the child with encopresis can become the scapegoat for more extensive psychological dysfunction in the family. These families should be referred to a competent therapist familiar with the management of this kind of problem.

Identifying the factors affecting the normal development of continence and understanding the symbolic role played by the symptom of encopresis can be instrumental in planning treatment. Major upheavals in the child's life (death in the family, separation of parents, remarriage and relation with the extended family, birth of a sibling) can be responsible for antisocial behavior, displaced anger, and regression, and can only be corrected by proper intervention.

Cases where complex psychopathology underlies the encopresis are much more difficult to manage and require a team approach. Unfortunately, the number of therapists who are experienced in the management of encopretic children and their families is small, so that in many communities, the pediatrician or general practitioner will have to assume the main role in directing the care. Experimenting with methods based on charting and rewarding the child for accident-free periods can be useful sometimes and is a way of involving the child and reinforcing his successes.

## LAXATIVES

Occasionally, it will be necessary to stimulate the intestine with the use of a laxative. This is often the case when the child is being conditioned to develop new toilet habits or when chronic dilatation has resulted in a functional mega-rectum or megacolon. In these situations, an element of colonic atony is present and needs to be corrected; otherwise, prevention of reimpaction can be difficult. Familiarity with laxatives of various types is useful clinically, and enables sensible titration of the dosage and realistic expectation of their effects.

The most powerful cathartics are believed to act through inhibition of electrolyte and water absorption in the intestine and/or stimulation of peristalsis. In animal models, some laxatives can also be shown to stimulate potassium excretion in the colon. Recent work on the mechanism of action of osmotic laxatives, such as magnesium citrate or sodium phosphate, suggest that their effects are mediated through stimulation of gut hormones or stimulation of peristalsis, and not merely as the effect of physical equilibration of fluid toward the hypertonic lumen. Much needs to be learned about the simple and time-honored remedies used for catharsis.

The most commonly used laxatives are described below.

### Bulking Agents

Derivatives of psyllium or methylcellulose are dehydrated to prepare a powder with high hydrophilic properties. Chemically they are natural or synthetic polysaccharides, and their mode of action is thought to be related to stimulation of peristalsis by the increase in diameter of the bowel after hydrating and swelling. Interestingly, some of these agents have been tried in the management of certain chronic diarrheas, perhaps on the premise of nonspecific absorption of toxins or bile acids.

Many preparations are available in the market, the major differences among them being their solubility, taste, salt and calorie content, and convenience of dosage. It is important to encourage drinking after each dose to prevent obstipation or bezoar formation. Most preparations need to be ingested immediately after being dissolved in 6–8 oz of water. If left in the glass for too long, they gel and become very unpalatable and less effective. For this reason, they are not very suitable for use in younger children who tend to fuss and procrastinate in front of medicines.

Effects of bulking agents are seen after 1 or 2 days of use. Initial changes can be seen after 12 hours. Titration is not difficult and can be aimed at one to three soft movements a day. Use for more than a couple of weeks is difficult in children due to taste fatigue and the general messiness of administration.

## Osmotic Laxatives

Also called saline cathartics, these nonabsorbable salts draw increased volumes of water to the lumen and, as mentioned before, can also stimulate peristalsis and promote mass emptying.

The most commonly used ones contain magnesium salts (sulfate, citrate, or hydroxide) or polyethylene glycol (GoLYTELY). The latter preparation is useful for colonic cleanup at short notice, i.e., prior to proctoscopy, colonoscopy, or barium enema. Six to eight ounces of magnesium citrate taken the night before (in the average 7- to 10-year-old), will consistently induce stooling 3–5 hours later. One common complaint is crampy abdominal pain. This is rarely severe.

## Colonic Stimulants

Three major groups of compounds are included under this heading.

Anthraquinones (Examples: Cascara, Senna). — Derived from certain plants and chemically complex glycosides, the anthraquinones inhibit water absorption and stimulate peristalsis. They are reliable and habit-forming laxatives. Main side effects are excessive purgation with electrolyte abnormalities, intestinal cramps and, if used for prolonged periods of time, decreased muscle tone in the colon. Their effect usually takes place 4–6 hours after administration. Because of the stimulatory effects on peristalsis, they can be useful in chronic functional constipation with atony. During the period of retraining, these laxatives can enhance colonic sensation and sigmoid segmentation.

Diphenylmethanes (Examples: Phenolphthalein, Bisacodyl). — Their pharmacology is similar to the anthraquinones, producing fluid accumulation in the intestine and stimulating peristalsis. Bisacodyl is administered in enteric coated preparations because of its irritating properties. Those same properties make it suitable for use in suppository form. Dulcolax is a popular form of bisacodyl. Proctitis can result from prolonged use.

Hydroxy-Fatty Acids. — The prototype for this group of laxatives is castor oil, and its active factor is ricinoleic oil. A powerful membrane irritant, it has been shown to produce active secretion of water and also to affect electrolyte transport. In addition, it has damaging effects on cellular membranes and increases permeability. Castor oil should not be used in children, and for that matter, probably neither in adults.

## BIBLIOGRAPHY

1. Schnarfer L, Kumar MAC, White JJ: Differentiation and management of incontinence and constipation problems in children. *Surg Clin North Am* 1970; 50(4):895–905.

2. Barr RG, Levine MD, Wilkinson RH, et al: Chronic and occult stool retention: A clinical tool for its evaluation in school-aged children. *Clin Pediatr* 1978; 18(11):674–686.
3. Levine MD: Children with encopresis: A descriptive analysis. *Pediatrics* 1975; 56:412.

# 11

# Gastrointestinal Bleeding

Not all that is red or black is blood, but when a child vomits what appears to be blood or passes maroon, tarry, or bright red stools, fright is the parent's immediate reaction, and medical attention is usually quickly sought.

Confirming the presence of blood and assessing the severity of the bleeding are the priorities of the practitioner. Prompt referral to a hospital will be indicated in the majority of cases of documented upper GI bleed, while passage of blood per rectum will in many cases be of a less emergent nature.

## DEFINITIONS

*Hematemesis* refers to the vomiting of blood, and it can be bright red or dark, depending on whether there has been sufficient time for the hemoglobin to be acid-denatured in the stomach. *Coffee ground* vomitus is a graphic term that describes this darker appearing hemoglobin. Hematemesis results from lesions in the esophagus, stomach, and sometimes from the duodenum. Bleeding from the nasopharynx and oral structures (gums, tongue, or teeth) can be inapparent and can present as hematemesis. Blood is a relatively potent emetic. Blood passed per rectum can be bright red — *hematochezia* — or tarry black and sticky with a very characteristic smell — *melena*. Hematochezia usually results from lesions in the colon or terminal ileum while melena is typical of sources above the ligament of Treitz and upper small intestine. Because blood is also a cathartic, profuse upper intestinal bleed can present as hematochezia; on the other hand, blood can become dark if it remains in the colon for a long enough time.

## CONFIRMING THE PRESENCE OF BLOOD

One of the first considerations is to determine whether blood is indeed present in the vomiting or stool. Food coloring added to cereals, drinks, medications, gelatine desserts, ketchup, and other tomato dishes can be deceivingly similar to blood, especially to an anxious parent. Dark vegetables, bismuth compounds such as found in Pepto-Bismol, iron-fortified cereals, or medicinal iron supplements can turn the stools black. Confirmation of the presence of hemoglobin in body fluids can be accomplished with readily available test tablets or slides. This is of particular importance in the workup of suspected occult bleeding as a source of unexplained anemia.

Identification of heme products is based on the interaction of peroxidase activity found in hemoglobin and various reagents. Among the most commonly used are *guaiac* (as found in the Hemoccult II slides), *orthotoluidin* (Hematest tablets) or *benzidine*. Because the benzidine reaction is very sensitive, a high rate of false positive results limits its usefulness. Guaiac-based tests are most reliable, but still have a false positive rate of 1%–2%. High doses of vitamin C will produce false negative guaiac tests, and diets containing radishes, turnips, and horseradish will cause false positives due to their high content of peroxidase. Hemoglobin in red meat will also result in a false positive test. Developing of the slides with the peroxide-containing reagent should be done within 3–6 days. None of the tests are 100% specific, and sensitivity varies depending on whether the reaction takes place in acid (gastric contents) or neutral pH. Newer products such as the Gastroccult have improved the sensitivity for detecting GI bleeding in vomitus or gastric contents. Several consecutive stools should be sampled when searching for occult bleeding, since polyps and other lesions can bleed only intermittently. In the adult, loss of more than 2.5 cc of blood per day is considered abnormal. Recently, actual quantitation of the hemoglobin present per gram of stool has emerged as an accurate diagnostic test mainly used in adults for carcinoma screening purposes.*

## HEMODYNAMIC EFFECTS OF BLEEDING

Once we have determined that the child is losing blood, the severity of the bleeding and its hemodynamic effects need to be assessed as accurately as possible. These effects are more prominent when the patient has bled acutely.

*Hemoquant: SmithKline Diagnostics.

Slow GI bleeds can be tolerated remarkably well and might present only with tiredness, pallor, dizziness, or fainting. Remembering that the circulating blood volume of a child is about 80–85 ml/kg and that orthostatic changes appear when there has been more than 20% reduction of blood volume, one can roughly appraise the severity of the bleed and the need for intensive care. Orthostatic changes are present when the pulse accelerates by 20 beats/minute or the systolic blood pressure drops by 10 mm Hg when the patient's position is changed from recumbent to seating.

## MOST COMMON ETIOLOGIES OF GI BLEEDING ACCORDING TO AGE GROUPS

In the neonatal period, one of the most common reasons for hematemesis or melena is the ingestion of maternal blood during delivery. Because fetal hemoglobin is more resistant to alkali denaturation than adult hemoglobin, a test based on this property will help identify the source of the hemoglobin. The *Apt test* can be done at the bedside and requires a 1% solution (0.25 M) of sodium hydroxide. The stool or vomitus is diluted 1:10 in water (to effect hemolysis), and after filtration or centrifugation, the hydroxide is added to the clear supernatant. A brown color reflects denatured maternal hemoglobin while dissolved fetal hemoglobin unaffected by the alkali will appear pink.

Another less commonly recognized source of apparent bleeding is from inadvertent ingestion of blood during breast feeding. At times, the mother is not even aware of a crack in her nipple, and it is surprising how much blood can be swallowed by a hungry nursing infant.

In the nursery, more serious bleeding results from *hemorrhagic disease*, seen much less commonly since the widespread prophylactic administration of vitamin K. A bleeding diathesis can be precipitated by antibiotic use and feeding of formulas low in vitamin K. It is also more likely to occur in exclusively breast-fed infants. The vitamin K-dependent clotting factors include prothrombin (II), proconvertin (VII), plasma thromboplastin component (IX), and Stuart-Prower factor (X). Vitamin K deficiency can develop in conditions resulting in fat malabsorption and steatorrhea such as cystic fibrosis and cholestatic syndromes.

Additional hemorrhagic disorders to be ruled out in the bleeding infant include disseminated intravascular coagulation and von Willebrand's disease. The first is often a complication of gram negative septicemia and endotoxemia, while von Willebrand's disease is an inherited defect involving platelet adhesiveness and abnormal factor VIII concentrations and function. Special coagulation studies, measuring fibrin degradation products, platelet function, and the response of factor VIII to plasma infusions are necessary to accurately diagnose these conditions.

Bleeding diathesis can result in hematemesis from diffuse gingival and gastric erosions. Subcutaneous hemorrhages and intraventricular bleeds can be major complications.

*Necrotizing enterocolitis* presents with GI bleeding in all but the mildest forms. Bleeding can range from faintly heme positive gastric aspirates to massive hematochezia. Necrotizing enterocolitis (NEC) must be suspected in any infant (particularly if premature and stressed) who develops apnea/bradycardia, hypo- or hyperthermia, decreased gastric emptying, abdominal distention, or heme positive stools.

The entire bowel can be affected, but it occurs more often in the right colon and terminal ileum. Intestinal ischemia resulting from arteriolar thrombi, mucosal ulcerations, and hemorrhage into the submucosa can rapidly progress to partial or total pneumonatosis intestinalis, perforation, and bowel gangrene. Healing can be complete or result in strictures (often multiple) in over one-third of the patients.

The etiology of NEC has remained elusive but is most likely multifactorial. The role of hypertonic formulas high in carbohydrates that cannot be completely digested and absorbed and might promote bacterial overgrowth has been implicated in several outbreaks. Nurseries in which enteral feedings of isotonic formulas are advanced very slowly report a much lower incidence of NEC. Bacterial toxins and enteroinvasive organisms have also been involved in epidemics. Breast milk appears to be protective. Treatment consists of nasogastric decompression intravenous antibiotics, close radiologic and clinical monitoring to diagnose perforation, and surgery if this has occurred or if no improvement follows intensive supportive therapy.

## Anatomical Abnormalities

Midgut volvulus, arteriovenous malformations, and duplication cysts of the intestine can all present with bleeding in the neonatal period, sometimes with catastrophic severity. The infant will have signs of intestinal obstruction and appear ill, and bleeding resulting from gangrenous bowel is ominous. Bleeding from esophageal varices is not common in the neonatal period but has been described in children with severe cytomegalovirus neonatal hepatitis. This diagnosis will be suggested by the presence of a jaundiced neonate showing signs of hepatic decompensation (ascites, bleeding). Gastric and duodenal ulcers can occur in the stressed and (much less commonly) nonstressed neonates. Hematochezia can result from brisk bleedings.

## Rectal Bleeding in the Neonate

Swallowed maternal blood is probably the most common reason for rectal bleeding in an otherwise healthy appearing infant. Perianal irritation and excoriations can result in small amounts of occult or streaky bleeding. Fissures can develop at any age and can also result in streaks of blood. The rectal mucosa at this young age is delicate, and if *nodular lymphoid hyperplasia* is present, friability can be sufficient to cause superficial bleeding with straining or passage of diarrheal stools. Anal and rectal fissures are often exquisitely painful and can be the underlying reason for irritability and distressed crying. Irritability due to painful defecation can be mistakenly confused with esophagitis and GE reflux since a straining and crying infant is more prone to vomit and the gastrocolic reflex will result in a bowel movement at the time of feedings.

Anal fissures are apparent by gently spreading the buttocks. The shiny mucosa will most often occur posteriorly or a small skin tag ("sentinel pile") might be present between the anus and the perineum. Rectal fissures can be felt by digital palpation with a well-lubricated glove. Use of the pinky is recommended for infants lest a fissure be produced by the examination itself. Examination with a test tube is to be discouraged. Accidental breaks can occur with serious consequences, and visibility is difficult in the best of circumstances. A pediatric proctoscope can readily detect the fissuring and provide additional important information about the rectal mucosa, and show evidence of generalized involvement with inflammation or the appearance of blood above the reach of the instrument. If a pediatric proctoscope is not available, an otoscope with a medium-sized speculum can at least provide excellent visualization of a limited segment of the anal canal and give bright illumination for inspection of the perianal area.

Loose stools mixed in with blood should raise the possibility of milk-induced or postantibiotic colitis. A stool smear will confirm inflammation, polymorphonuclear leukocytes and Charcot-Leyden crystals (remnants of eosinophils). A much more serious cause of colitis and bloody diarrhea in the neonate is the enteritis associated with Hirschsprung's disease. Prompt recognition is imperative since mortality is high. Colonic dilatation, toxemia, and shock can develop rapidly. The underlying aganglionosis is at times unsuspected at this stage. Aggressive treatment of fluid and electrolyte disturbances, rectal decompression and irrigations, antibiotics, and nasogastric intubation are necessary to avert progression to perforation and irreversible shock.

## Bleeding in the First 5 Years of Life

Upper gastrointestinal bleeding in this age group is most frequently due to esophagitis, gastritis, or peptic ulcers. If the bleeding develops after forceful vomiting, a *Mallory-Weiss tear* has to be suspected. The longitudinal laceration occurs most frequently in the esophagogastric junction, and profuse bleeding can ensue from disruption of vessels in the submucosa. Bleeding from a Mallory-Weiss tear can also present as melena. Diagnosis is made endoscopically, and management is conservative in most cases, unless bleeding goes on unabated.

*Foreign bodies* can damage the tongue, pharynx, esophagus, or stomach. Initial bleeding can subside shortly after the ingestion only to reappear when erosion into a vessel or perforation develop.

*Enteric duplication cysts* containing ectopic gastric mucosa can be present along the mesenteric side of any part of the intestinal tract. Their lumen can be communicating with the lumen of the intestine, in which case erosion of adjacent mucosa can result in bleeding. Cysts can also be leading points for intussusceptions or result in intestinal obstruction. *Intestinal tumors* are a much less common source of hematemesis.

## Rectal Bleeding

Rectal bleeding will accompany bacterial infections, protein allergy, or localized rectal lesions. The clinical presentation will give useful information and will help determine the most likely diagnosis.

Painless bleeding, typically maroon colored alternating with bright red, will most likely result from a *Meckel's diverticulum* or a polyp. The diverticulum is a remnant of the omphalomesenteric duct which connected the yolk sac to the intestine (Fig 11–1). It is always on the antimesenteric border of the ileum, usually within a foot of the ileocecal valve. One-third of the diverticula contain gastric or pancreatic mucosa, and it is for this reason that bleeding occurs. The erosions are either at the base of the diverticulum or in the ileum adjacent to it. When a large vessel is involved, the bleeding can be severe. Bleeding from a Meckel's diverticulum can occur at any age, but is more common in the first 2 years of life. Other complications associated with this anomaly are intussusception, volvulus around a long omphalomesenteric band, bowel gangrene, and, rarely, diverticulitis with or without a foreign body. The diagnosis is most frequently made on clinical grounds since radiological demonstration of the lesion is rare. The parietal cells in gastric epithelium concentrate technetium 99m pertechnetate and can help identify the diverticulum if enough ectopic mucosa is present in it. A negative test is never considered a sufficient reason not to explore a patient in whom the diagnosis is strongly suspected.

*Colonic polyps* (inflammatory, juvenile polyps) are benign lesions in their majority, and often present as painless rectal bleeding. Male children in the age group 2 to 6 years are most affected. In the majority of cases, the polyp is single and autoamputates by trauma or by infarction of the feeding vessels at the pedicle. Luckily, 90% of the polyps arise in the rectosigmoid and are easily visualized, even with a rigid scope.

Other colonic polyps appear later and can be associated with familiar syndromes inherited in most of the cases as autosomal dominant and important because of the extremely high risk of malignancy. In *familial colonic polyposis*,

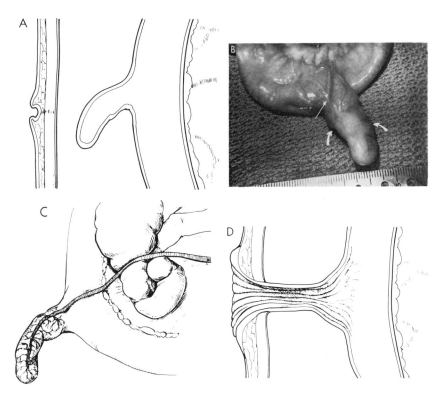

**FIG 11–1.**
**A**, Meckel's diverticulum remains unattached in the majority (74%) of cases. **B**, typical appearance of Meckel's diverticulum at celiotomy. It arises from the anti-mesenteric border of the ileum, usually within 100 cm of the ileocecal junction, and is of approximately the same caliber as the ileum. The majority of symptomatic Meckel's diverticula (75%) contain heterotopic elements (most commonly gastric mucosa) that can often be seen and palpated on external examination, as in this case. The pale appearance (distal to *curved arrows*) represents heterotopic gastric mucosa within the diverticulum. Ease of palpability can be correlated with an increased measured area of gastric mucosa in the diverticulum. The blood supply is seen continuing from beneath the ileal serosa into the body of the diverticulum (*straight arrow*). **C**, the blood supply is derived from the paired vitelline (omphal-omesenteric) arteries that pass on either side of the mesentery to ramify over the yolk sac. The left vitelline artery normally disappears, while the proximal part of the right vessel becomes the superior mesenteric artery. Its distal segment persists as an end artery of this parent vessel and supplies remnants of the vitelline duct. The vitelline (omphalomesenteric) vessels usually terminate in the diverticulum but can continue to the abdominal wall (*dotted line*). **D**, in the latter instance, the vitelline vessels may also persist as a fibrous cord connecting ileum to the umbilicus after complete involution of the diverticulum. This can set the stage for intestinal obstruction. (From Welch KJ, Randolph JG, Ravitch MM, et al: *Pediatric Surgery*, ed 4. Chicago, Year Book Medical Publishers, 1986. Used by permission.)

the lesions are adenomatous polyps while in Gardner's syndrome, adenomas are found in association with soft tissue tumors, osteomas, and epidermal cysts. In both of these conditions, prophylactic colectomy is indicated. The possibility of an ileoanal endorectal pullthrough now offers a fair chance for continence. Screening of all family members by means of colonoscopy or air contrast barium enemas must be done diligently.

In contrast, the intestinal polyps in the Peutz-Jeghers syndrome are located mainly in the small intestine. Pathologically, the polyps are hamartomas, and only in rare instances has malignant transformation been reported. The typical skin lesions are pigmented macules present in the oral and labial mucosa. Clinical presentation includes anemia, recurrent abdominal pains, and intermittent intestinal obstruction with intussusception and melena. The pigmented lesions appear in late childhood and early adolescence.

## Bleeding in the Older Child and Adolescent

Upper gastrointestinal bleeding in this age group is most frequently due to *peptic ulcer disease* (duodenal and gastric), gastritis, and esophageal varices. Peptic ulcer disease is more common in males. Melena can be the presenting symptom in half of the patients. Hematemesis or hematochezia can be followed by hypotension and shock, and abdominal pain can be prominent. *Variceal bleeding* is usually painless and profuse, and fortunately is well tolerated initially. Even in the presence of esophageal varices, another source of bleeding (gastric varices, duodenal ulcer) can be found in about 40% of patients, and the exact source of an upper GI bleed can now be accomplished in most cases by the use of fiberoptic endoscopy. Therapeutic intervention is also possible, whether laser or bipolar coagulation of bleeding vessels or with injection of sclerosing solutions to esophageal varices.

Variceal bleeding can sometimes be the initial presentation of portal hypertension, usually when the underlying etiology is extrahepatic portal hypertension. *Cavernous transformation of the portal vein*, a complication of omphalitis or umbilical vein catheterization, and *congenital hepatic fibrosis* are the most common entities. Fortunately, hepatic parenchymal function is well preserved in both instances, and results after portosystemic shunting are satisfactory. Subtle intellectual changes can occur after shunts even in this population, so that the long-term results are not so clear. But portal hypertension associated with cirrhosis has a much poorer prognosis, and hepatic function tends to deteriorate after most shunting procedures. Jaundice and/or ascites are usually present by the time bleeding from varices occurs.

The association of intestinal and renal manifestations can be found in the *hemolytic uremic syndrome* and *Henoch-Schönlein purpura*. Vasculitis is responsible for edema of the bowel, rectal bleeding, intestinal obstruction, and perforation. In Henoch-Schönlein purpura, the intestinal manifestations can precede the rash which is initially urticarial and later turns ecchymotic and purpuric. Buttocks and lower extremities are preferentially involved. Hematuria and proteinuria can be prominent or microscopic, and the renal involvement ultimately determines the prognosis, since some patients can progress to renal failure. Intestinal bleeding can be severe and recurrent, and intussusception can develop, with edematous loops of bowel as the lead point. Close observation is necessary to ward off ischemic necrosis and perforation. Symptoms improve on steroid therapy. Prednisone 1–2 mg/kg/day can result in dramatic resolution of the abdominal pains, which can be severe. Steroids and platelet antiaggregants seem to improve the prognosis.

The hemolytic uremic syndrome can be accompanied by an ischemic colitis presenting with diarrhea and rectal bleeding. There is oliguria and pallor, and the youngster or child can appear quite ill with abdominal guarding, vomiting, and lethargy. Intussusception needs to be ruled out, and prognosis is dependent on the renal lesion. Familial forms have been described and have a worse prognosis. A viral etiology has been postulated, and clustering of cases in geographical areas suggests an infectious agent. There is laboratory evidence of microangiopathic hemolysis and later azotemia. Abnormal liver function tests reflect involvement of the liver by the vasculitic process. Management is supportive and intensive, since recovery of renal function is possible even in the face of prolonged renal failure.

## SUGGESTIONS FOR THE INVESTIGATION OF GI BLEEDING

After the initial evaluation of the hemodynamic stability of the patient and as the immediate measures for adequate venous access are instituted, as much information as possible is gathered on pertinent points in the history. A preliminary differential diagnosis is sketched based on the nature and amount of the bleed, age of the patient, and prior clinical features: fever, vomiting, pain, decreased urine output, diarrhea, mental changes, skin lesions, etc.

At the time of venous catheter placement, blood is obtained for a complete count, including platelets, coagulation profile, SMA-12 or similar liver and kidney function profile, and a type and crossmatch.

Even if the suspected source is esophageal varices, no harm will be done if a nasogastric tube is inserted. This should be one of the first steps in the diagnostic approach of the patient with GI bleeding, whether it presents as hematochezia or melena or more obviously, as hematemesis. Gastric bleeding can sometimes present as hematochezia when transit time is rapid. The NG tube should be a sump tube with multiple holes, and lubrication should be generous.

Finding clots of blood, coffee ground material, or fresh blood suggests an esophageal or gastric source, but blood from the duodenum can sometimes flow retrogradely and appear in the aspirates as well.

If blood is found in the stomach, repeated lavage with saline will help assess the briskness of the bleed. Recent studies suggest that the old practice of using ice-cold lavage solution is probably not any more effective than using it at room temperature. Of greater concern is the finding of abnormal coagulation function induced by the iced solution and changes in blood flow not clearly beneficial. Ice-cold lavage will slowly join other long lasting and firmly believed medical traditions abandoned for more rational and experimentally proven ones.

If the bleeding does not subside after repeated lavage, the next step will depend on the severity of the bleed. If the rate is exsanguinating, urgent surgery might be the only way to control the situation, and no time should be lost in transferring an unstable patient to nuclear scanning or to the angiography suite.

If bleeding continues and the patient is hemodynamically stable (transfused if necessary), upper endoscopy offers the best yield in identifying the source. In the infant or young child, endoscopy needs sometimes to be done under general anesthesia with proper monitoring. Specific treatment can then be planned based on the findings, whether it be sclerotherapy of esophageal varices or pharmacological therapy of gastritis or ulcers. The presence of an arterial "bleeder" at the center of an ulcer usually portends a high risk of recurrence, and the surgical consult should be prepared to intervene if massive bleeding recurs. If experienced intervention radiologists are available, arteriography can identify and help control bleeding from AV malformations and other sources.

If the bleeding has ceased at the time of lavage, an upper GI series (double contrast, if possible) should be done. Identification of a source should then be treated. If varices are suggested by the physical evidence of portal hypertension and by the radiographic findings of the study, endoscopy for confirmation of the diagnosis and for initiation of sclerotherapy is indicated.

When the nasogastric aspirates are negative and a lower GI source is likely, a scout film of the abdomen helps identify obstruction. A barium enema might identify the location of the obstruction and, in the case of an intussusception, will be curative in most instances.

If there is no obstruction, a proctosigmoidoscopy (flexible, if available) will distinguish between generalized oozing from colitis or suggest a discrete lesion. Often, a polyp or part of its stalk is found during this simple procedure. A Tc-pertechnate scan should be ordered if a source is not identified and a Meckel's diverticulum is suspected.

If the bleeding is intermittent and severe and no sources are found after barium enema and colonoscopy, arteriography should be planned if labelled red cell scanning fails to document a bleeding site. A bleeding rate of at least 0.5 cc/min is needed to permit visualization by angiography.

The infusion of vasopressin intravenously shunts blood away from the splanchnic circulation and tends to control bleeding from varices, gastritis, or other unidentified sources. Close monitoring of serum electrolytes (hyponatremia), cardiovascular status, and peripheral circulation is mandatory.

In summary, after stabilizing the patients vital signs, nasogastric aspiration becomes the first, simplest, and most revealing diagnostic step. Once the source is identified (endoscopy, contrast studies, nuclear medicine, arteriography), the therapeutic options need to be adjusted to the particular case.

## Peptic Ulcer

The gastric and duodenal mucosa of children is not immune to damage by pepsin, acid, and chemicals. Factors determining the formation of a superficial erosion or a deeper ulcer are not fully understood, but the importance of hydrochloric acid and pepsin is well established (''no acid, no ulcer''). Also important are mucosal protective factors mediated by prostaglandins and the quality and quantity of the mucinous secretions lining the epithelial cells. Normal perfusion and oxygenation are also protective, and disruption of cellular integrity often occurs during severe hypovolemia and hypoxia, especially in the newborn.

### Physiological Aspects

Gastric acid is produced by the *parietal cells*, found in higher density in the area of the antrum of the stomach. The parietal cell mass is believed to be high in newborns, and its control is under the influence of neurohormonal factors (vagal, gastrin, other).

Despite the hypergastrinemia found in newborns, acid production is lower at that time and does not reach adult levels until about 6 months of age. A decrease in the number of gastrin receptors or an insensitivity to gastrin has been postulated. *Gastrin* is released by vagal stimulation after gastric dilatation and by certain peptones and amino acids in the diet, as well as by caffeine, aminophyllin, alcohol, and calcium salts. *Histamine* released from mast cells closely apposed to blood vessels under the mucosa and synthesized in *oxyntic cells* is also a powerful stimulator of acid production.

The maximal secretory capacity after stimulation with a histamine analog (Histalog) or pentagastrin is commonly used to assess gastric secretion. Unfortunately, there is a great deal of overlapping between the basal and maximal acid outputs in patients with peptic ulcer disease of the stomach and controls. In general, maximal and peak acid output tends to be higher in patients with primary duodenal ulcers. Similarly, postprandial serum gastrin levels in patients with peptic disease is not different from controls. Serum gastrin is elevated in the *Zollinger-Ellison syndrome* and in some hypercalcemic states. *Pepsinogen I* also originates in the oxyntic cells in the stomach and, according to recent studies, its concentration in the serum appears to be higher in some patients with duodenal ulcers.

Predisposition for duodenal ulcers is a familiar trait. Fathers of children with primary duodenal ulcers often also give a positive ulcer history. There is a threefold increased incidence in identical twins. The HLA-B5 and BW phenotypes were thought to be found with increased frequency in patients with duodenal ulcers, but more extensive experience does not confirm those findings. There is an excess of blood group O in patients developing duodenal ulcers in their 30s.

Much less clear is the association between a personality profile and the risk for ulcer disease. Psychosocial adaptation problems, reaction to feelings and coping mechanisms for frustration, dependency, and aggressiveness have been shown as areas of differences between children with ulcer disease and age-matched controls.

Peptic ulcer disease is not a common reason for hospitalization (2–5 of 10,000 pediatric admissions), but the true prevalence of these disorders is unknown. Given the nonspecific nature of the symptoms in infants and young children, we are most probably underestimating its occurrence.

### Clinical Presentation

The younger the child, the higher the likelihood of peptic ulcer disease presenting with a serious complication: perforation, bleeding, shock, abdominal distention, or high obstruction. In the newborn, ulcers are more common in the stomach, and perforations occur close to the greater curve. As previously mentioned, gastric ulcers in the newborn are more common following a stressful delivery, prematurity, sepsis, hypoglycemia, or hypoxia. They also occur in infants with none of these risk factors. There is no sex predilection.

Up to the preschool years, vomiting is the most common symptom. Decreased oral intake, anorexia, weight loss, and irritability should always be carefully assessed. These symptoms can persist for months since the diagnosis and specific treatment is often not even considered. A high index of suspicion is necessary when dealing with the child with poor feeding habits, excessive crying, or vomiting. Anemia or bleeding, rather than perforation, is the more common serious complication in this age group.

In children older than 6 years, pain is the most common presenting symptom. Only one-third of the patients will give a history of "typical" pain, i.e., hunger-related, improved by eating, nocturnal. The location of the pain tends to become more epigastric as the child gets older and is able to express and localize discomfort. Periumbilical pain, early morning, and postprandial symptoms are also common. Hematemesis or melena occur in half of the patients in this age group. Boys are almost four times more involved than girls.

## Secondary Ulcers

Ulcers occurring in the context of severe disease or associated with stress are termed secondary. Interestingly, they are not always associated with hypergastrinemia or hyperacidity. Postulated mechanisms have included changes in membrane permeability, steroid-mediated effects on gastric mucus, and increased histamine release. Special names have been coined for the ulcers developing during head trauma, surgery, or CNS infection (*Cushing's ulcers*), or following burns (*Curling's ulcers*). Their etiology remains unclear, although increased acid secretion has been demonstrated in Cushing's ulcers.

### Diagnosis

Peptic ulcer is the major diagnostic consideration when a child presents with GI bleeding, either hematemesis or melena. When the bleeding is massive, as it tends to be, aggressive management is needed to stabilize the patient. Reassessment of the hemodynamic changes occurring as a result of the blood loss takes precedence in the evaluation. Surgical consultation is often indicated early on to prepare for eventual failure of medical therapy. A high index of suspicion helps diagnose peptic ulcer disease presenting with abdominal pain or vomiting.

### Differential Diagnosis

Major considerations in the differential diagnosis include gastroesophageal reflux with or without esophagitis, pancreatitis, inflammatory bowel disease, food intolerance, and gallbladder dysfunction.

Once the diagnosis is entertained, a number of investigations are available for its evaluation. Because of the atypical nature of the pain, the inconsistent association with meals, and the spontaneous improvement in the symptoms with unpredictable recurrences, the diagnosis can be very difficult at times. The presence of anemia, guaiac positive stools, and obviously blood-streaked vomitus will naturally prompt a more extensive workup.

The yield of an upper GI series in detecting gastric ulcers is half of an upper endoscopy, but the easiness of the procedure still makes it the examination of choice in the investigation of a child with suspected peptic ulcer disease. The sensitivity is somewhat better for duodenal ulcers. Using the double-contrast technique, mucosal definition is greatly enhanced and identification of the ulcer crater becomes more precise.

The diagnosis cannot be made on the basis of pyloric spasm seen during fluoroscopy. Prominent folds in the stomach or duodenum are sometimes suggestive but can often be seen in normal studies and do not constitute sufficient evidence of ulcer disease. Gastric outlet obstruction can be secondary to edema and deformity of the bulb, or can be a purely functional disorder. Superficial erosions can only be detected by direct observation.

Upper endoscopy can be done in children of all ages. New endoscopes are as small (or big) as a 14F tube and can be introduced without compromise to the airway. Sedation with meperidine and diazepam and Xylocaine spraying of the throat enable adequate examination with proper nursing care and monitoring. Endoscopy offers the highest yield for diagnosing gastritis and bleeding secondary ulcers. It is also indicated in the investigation of persistent symptoms despite adequate therapy or when mucosal irregularities detected radiologically remain unchanged after treatment.

*Treatment*

The mainstay of therapy of peptic ulcer disease in the absence of serious complications is the suppression of acid production or the neutralization of gastric acidity with antacids. Maintaining gastric pH above 4.0 inactivates pepsin and promotes healing.

Antacids. — Aluminum hydroxide is constipating while magnesium hydroxide is a cathartic. Products containing mixtures of both ingredients or alternating preparations are best tolerated. Dosage is empiric, and precise titration is only possible by frequent aspiration of gastric contents. One teaspoon to two tablespoons according to weight (approximately 0.5 cc/kg/dose) is given 1 and 3 hours after meals and at bedtime (some recommend hourly doses during the day and at bedtime). Additional doses are given as needed for breakthrough symptoms. Therapy is continued for 6 to 8 weeks.

H-2 Receptor Antagonists. — Both cimetidine (Tagamet) and ranitidine (Zantac) are powerful inhibitors of acid secretion, and for many have become the therapy of choice to treat peptic ulcers despite the fact that when properly given, H-2 antagonists and antacids are of comparable efficacy.

Reported experience with cimetidine in children is limited, but its safety for short-term use is widely recognized. Changes in mental status have only been described in the geriatric population. Gynecomastia has not been reported in children, and is only seen in prolonged therapy (much longer than 6 weeks). Idiosyncratic and allergic reactions (fever, rashes), thrombocytopenia, elevated creatinine, and hepatic abnormalities have been reported. Overall, experience suggests that cimetidine is a safe drug for the management of ulcers in children. Usual dosage is 5–10 mg/kg/dose, every 6 hours, last dose at bedtime. Advantages of ranitidine include longer duration of action requiring 12-hour dosage and reportedly less side effects. Experience in pediatric patients is limited, and careful administration is necessary if this drug is chosen.

Sucralfate. — This recently introduced product is a complex of magnesium hydroxide and sulfated sucrose. It does not get absorbed and seems to exert its effect locally by binding to the exudate of the ulcer and perhaps by preventing back diffusion of hydrogen ions. Sucralfate also adsorbs bile acids and inactivates pepsin. Experience in adults has been favorable when used an hour before meals and at bedtime. The 1-gm tablets are large for use in young children, and a liquid form is not available. Its role in the long-term management of peptic ulcer disease or peptic esophagitis in adults and children has not been established.

Diet. — It will come as a surprise to most patients and their parents to hear that there is no need for drastic dietary changes. There is no evidence that a bland diet influences ulcer healing. Drinking citrus juices will sometimes exacerbate dyspepsia, and any other associations between food and symptoms should be assessed on an individual basis. Since food itself stimulates acid production, frequent small meals should be avoided. Three meals a day is preferable.

Following an upper GI bleed, diet should be initially light to test gastric emptying and give a chance for normal function to return. Alcohol ingestion should be discouraged in the adolescent. Smoking delays ulcer healing and should also be avoided. Of course, aspirin and other nonsteroidal anti-inflammatory medications should not be used. Acetaminophen does not adversely influence ulcer healing and can be safely used in these patients.

## BIBLIOGRAPHY

1. Ament ME, Christie DL: Upper gastrointestinal fiberoptic endoscopy in pediatric patients. *Gastroenterology* 1977; 72:1244.
2. Cox K, Ament ME: Upper gastrointestinal bleeding in children and adolescents. *Pediatrics* 1979; 63:408.
3. Eidelman A, Inwood RJ: Necrotizing enterocolitis and enteral feedings. *Am J Dis Child* 1980; 134:553.
4. Fromm D: Salicylate and gastric mucosal damage. *Pediatrics* 1978; 62:938.
5. Gryboski JD: The role of endoscopy in upper gastrointestinal bleeding in infants and children. *Dig Dis Sci* 1981; 26:175.
6. Kleigman RM, Fanaroff A: Neonatal necrotizing enterocolitis: A nine-year experience. *Am J Dis Child* 1971; 135:603.
7. Parikh N, Sebring E, Polesky H: Evaluation of blood gastric fluid from newborn infants. *J Pediatr* 1979; 94:967.
8. Raffensperger JG, Luck SR: Gastrointestinal bleeding in children. *Surg Clin North Am* 1976; 36:413.
9. Schullinger JN, Mollit DL, Vinocur CD, et al: Neonatal necrotizing enterocolitis. *Am J Dis Child* 1981; 135:612.
10. Upadhyaya K, Barwich K, Fishaut M, et al: The importance of nonrenal involvement in the hemolytic uremic syndrome. *Pediatrics* 1980; 65:115.
11. Nuss D, Lynn H: Peptic ulceration in children. *Surg Clin North Am* 1971; 51:945.

# 12

# Inflammatory Bowel Disease

As the incidence and prevalence of inflammatory bowel disease (IBD) continues to increase throughout the world, the chances are high that a busy pediatrician will be faced with this diagnosis 4 to 5 times a year. Depending on the demographics of the practice, this figure can easily be twice as much.

It is important to remember the particular ways in which IBD can present in the pediatric population, since referrals are often made to endocrinologists or even psychiatrists when children and adolescents offer vague complaints of abdominal pains, anorexia, or failure to grow.

It is also important to understand that the term IBD is reserved for ileitis and colitis of unknown etiology and that a diagnosis is usually made after infection is ruled out by a careful history and repeated stool cultures. The differential diagnosis is presented in Table 12–1.

## ETIOLOGY

Unfortunately, we cannot yet answer with any degree of confidence one of the first questions parents ask when given the diagnosis of IBD. What causes this disease? Why does it run in the family? Why can't we cure it? How can we treat it effectively? What is the prognosis?

TABLE 12–1.
Differential Diagnosis of Inflammatory Bowel
Disease Involving the Colon

INFECTIONS
Bacterial
  *Shigella*
  *Salmonella*
  *Yersinia*
  *Campylobacter*
  Tuberculosis
  Gonorrhea
  *Staphylococcus*
Fungal
  Histoplasma
Protozoan
  Amebae
  Schistosoma

CLINICAL/PATHOLOGICAL ENTITIES
  Pseudomembranous (postantibiotics) colitis
  Ischemic colitis
  Uremic colitis
  Laxative abuse
  Familial polyposis syndromes
  Collagen vascular diseases
  Irritable bowel syndrome

Over the last 60 years, since Crohn, Oppenheimer, and Ginsburg described granulomatous ileitis, the similarities to intestinal tuberculosis were noted, but until now, the search for an infectious agent fulfilling Koch's four postulates has eluded scientists. Candidate agents have included viruses, wall-free (L-forms) bacteria, and mycobacteria. Interest in the latter has found renewed momentum since a slow-growing mycobacterium was discovered in intestinal material from patients with ileitis.

The immunological response of the host to any of the above mentioned infectious agents or to other antigens postulated to be present in the diet is probably of importance in explaining the chronicity of the inflammation. Activated lymphocytes homing on intestinal cells because the offending agent(s) share antigenic similarities, are likely vectors of the progressive and long lasting damage seen in IBD. Advances in immunology will undoubtedly provide a clearer picture of the cytopathic mechanisms involved. What it cannot answer at this time is whether those abnormal immunological responses are a cause of the disease or merely an abnormal response to a more basic and still elusive etiologic factor(s).

# CROHN'S DISEASE AND ULCERATIVE COLITIS

Both granulomatous inflammation and ulcerative colitis can be found in several members of the same family, but the clinical course, complications, and prognosis (particularly in respect to the risk of cancer) are very different. Only in a small minority of patients (less than 5%) will the diagnosis remain in doubt even after all investigations are completed. This is particularly the case in certain instances of Crohn's colitis where the disease remains superficial and biopsies do not provide pathological confirmation of granuloma formation. The difficulty is not one of mere academic interest, since the results of surgery and the treatment options are very different for these two conditions.

## Pathological Features

Pathologically, ulcerative colitis affects only the colon. Inflammation of the terminal ileum by incompetence of the ileocecal valve and reflux of bacteria and colonic contents ("backwash ileitis") is sometimes present, but the small intestine is never involved by the same process seen in the colon.

The hallmark of ulcerative colitis is the *crypt abscess*, clearly seen in suction biopsies obtained during colonoscopy. Acute inflammatory cells (polymorphonuclears), edema, hemorrhage, destruction and distortion of the mucous glands, and ulceration extend proximally from the rectum. In contrast with Crohn's colitis, rectal sparing is very unusual in ulcerative colitis, and the inflammation tends to be complete, circumferential, and without skip areas. Inflammation affects the mucosa, submucosa, and sometimes extends deep into the muscularis mucosa. Only in severe colitis, especially in association with toxic dilatation, does the inflammation reach the serosa, but the tendency of the intestinal loops to mat against each other is notoriously missing. As a result, when perforation occurs in ulcerative colitis, it tends to be a free perforation with massive peritoneal soiling. In contrast, in Crohn's disease, perforations tend to be confined as walled-off abscesses by thickened omental folds and mesenteric fat.

In Crohn's disease, inflammation is segmental and transmural. Pathologically, *granulomas* can be found in a third of the cases. Crypt abscesses can be indistinguishable from ulcerative colitis, and only clinical and radiological features allow making that distinction. Healing results in proliferation of connective tissue and scar formation. Narrowed areas can eventually lead to partial or complete obstruction. Linear ulcerations and deep scars result in the typical "cobblestoning" pattern often seen radiographically.

## Clinical Features

One third of the patients with IBD will have symptoms before adolescence. Although rare, well-documented cases of idiopathic ulcerative colitis and Crohn's disease have been described in infants and young children. In the majority of cases, onset of symptoms can be traced from age 9 through adolescence.

## Symptoms

The most common presenting symptoms are somewhat different in ulcerative colitis and Crohn's. A list is presented in Table 12–2. The most common are discussed below.

*Tenesmus*, the sensation of fecal urgency occurring after an evacuation, is most typically seen in ulcerative colitis, and is an important feature to be elicited during the history. It invariably means inflammation of the lower rectal area and anal canal, where rich sensory innervation is present. It occurs in other inflammatory conditions of the colon such as *Shigella* or *Salmonella* infection and, to judge by the infants' behavior, in milk-induced colitis as well.

*Diarrhea* is present in almost all patients with ulcerative colitis and in close to 85% of patients with Crohn's disease at the time of diagnosis. The stool in ulcerative colitis is a mixture of purulent exudate and mucoid material mixed in with bright red blood. In general, it is not of large volume. When large surface areas of the colon are involved, water reabsorption can be greatly affected and profuse diarrhea and incontinence can also develop. In severe cases, the patient might have 10–20 movements a day, nocturnal diarrhea being particularly distressing.

In Crohn's ileitis, diarrhea can be totally absent or can be severe and debilitating. Occult blood can be detected in a fair proportion of patients. Apparent rectal bleeding is less common. On the other hand, when bleeding does occur, it can be massive and life threatening because the source in those cases is usually a large vessel eroded by the inflammatory process, and not from diffuse, superficial erosions as seen in ulcerative colitis.

*Abdominal pain* is a presenting complaint in over three-fourths of the patients. The pattern and location of the pain is somewhat different in both conditions. In ulcerative colitis, it tends to be lower abdominal, along the descending colon and deep into the rectum. It is crampy, often severe, and occurs frequently in association with meals. Defecation brings relief (unless accompanied by severe tenesmus) until the next wave of colicky pains and urgency.

In Crohn's ileitis or ilecolitis, pain is more midabdominal or clearly localized to the right lower quadrant. Nausea, increased salivation, and anorexia accom-

TABLE 12–2.
Comparison of Presenting Symptoms in Ulcerative Colitis and Crohn's Disease

| SYMPTOMS | ULCERATIVE COLITIS | CROHN'S DISEASE |
|---|---|---|
| Abdominal pain | Often, with BMs | Very common |
| Diarrhea | Mostly severe | Less prominent or absent |
| Rectal bleeding | Very common | Rare |
| Anemia | Common | Common |
| Growth retardation | Little or none | Often marked |
| Extraintestinal manifestations | Uncommon | Common |

pany the general discomfort and can be symptoms of partial obstruction or interference with fecal flow due to strictures. Pain in Crohn's is also made worse by eating, a possible explanation for the decreased caloric intake usually found in patients with growth retardation. The patient or his family might not even be aware of the subtle appetite suppression caused by this learned response.

*Vomiting* is not very common in ulcerative colitis unless the disease is severe and extensive and the patient is debilitated and shows other signs of systemic involvement. In Crohn's disease, as mentioned before, nausea and vomiting are probably related to altered motility in areas of narrowing and increased gas production if bacterial overgrowth or malabsorption are present. Protracted vomiting, by then usually bilious or even fecal, is a sign of intestinal obstruction and needs urgent attention.

*Anorexia and weight loss* are much more common in Crohn's disease. Over 75% of patients with ileitis will present with weight loss, at times dramatic. In general, those patients look chronically ill, and indeed, malignancy needs to be ruled out early in the diagnostic workup. In ulcerative colitis, anorexia is a presenting symptom in half of the patients, and usually reflects disease activity. Anorexia can result from psychological depression in a youngster or adolescent overwhelmed by his or her disease. The constraints imposed by the continued need for medications, the physical side effects of steroids, tiredness, inability to compete, and fear of pain and incontinence are difficult obstacles placed in the already complex life of a growing adolescent.

*Fever*, be it cyclic, nocturnal, low grade, or spiking, is more commonly seen in Crohn's disease, where almost one-third of the patients will present with this symptom. Inflammatory bowel disease should always be considered in the evaluation of fever of unknown origin.

*Perianal lesions* are more commonly seen in Crohn's disease. Indolent ulcers and fissures can be found months or years before overt disease is detected. Skin tags, draining sinuses, perirectal abscesses, and fistulas can appear in the anal area. Unfortunately, fistula formation can occur between the intestine and any anatomical structure. Enterovesical, enterovaginal, enteroenteric, or enterocutaneous fistulas can develop spontaneously or following surgery and are typically difficult to treat and contribute significantly to the morbidity of Crohn's disease.

*Extraintestinal manifestations* are multisystemic and are another reflection of the generalized nature of this group of diseases. Skin, joints, eyes, mucosa, and the liver can be affected. A listing of the most common extraintestinal manifestations is presented in Table 12–3.

### Diagnosis

A suggested diagnostic algorithm for the evaluation of the patient presenting with a history of chronic diarrhea and other features suggestive of inflammatory bowel disease is presented in Figure 12–1. A high index of suspicion is necessary to diagnose Crohn's disease. A delay of 2–3 years is not unusual. Early signs

TABLE 12–3.
Extraintestinal Manifestations of Inflammatory
Bowel Disease

| Eyes | Uveitis/iritis |
|------|----------------|
| Skin | Pyoderma gangrenosum |
|      | Erythema nodosum |
| Joints | Clubbing |
|      | Arthritis |
|      | Spondylitis |
| Liver | Chronic active hepatitis |
|      | Cholangitis/biliary cirrhosis |
| Other | Amenorrhea |
|      | Growth retardation |

of the disease can be very subtle. When rectal bleeding is present, diagnosis is usually arrived at expeditiously because of the alarming nature of this complaint. Close attention to growth velocities is mandatory and any deceleration in linear growth or weight gain should be thoroughly evaluated. Self-limited conditions (particularly infectious) are ruled out, and the patient is referred to the gastroenterologist for further investigation.

In order of precedence, the workup will include, in addition to routine blood work (complete blood count, sedimentation rate, biochemical screen, amylase):

1. Bone age
2. Proctosigmoidoscopy with biopsy
3. X-rays studies
    a. Upper GI with small bowel follow-through
    b. Barium enema (double contrast, if possible)
4. Total flexible colonoscopy.

In the majority of cases, a firm diagnosis will be made when all studies have been completed. Microscopic identification of granulomas in the mucosal biopsies of rectum or colon cannot be obtained in more than 30% of ileal Crohn's so that the diagnosis of granulomatous inflammation, more often than not, rests on the constellation of abnormalities seen radiologically and on the clinical course (Fig 12–2).

## Treatment

Unfortunately, not much has changed in the management of inflammatory bowel disease in the past 4 decades. This is a reflection of our lack of understanding of the basic etiology of these diseases. The mainstays of therapy include: (1) adequate nutrition, (2) medications, and (3) emotional support to the patient and his or her family.

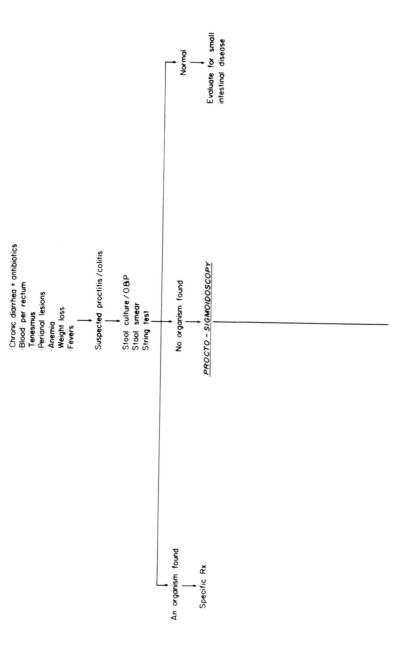

HISTORY OF:

-Chronic diarrhea ± antibiotics
-Blood per rectum
-Tenesmus
-Perianal lesions
-Anemia
-Weight loss
-Fevers

Suspected proctitis/colitis

Stool culture/O&P
Stool smear
String test

An organism found

Specific Rx

No organism found

*PROCTO-SIGMOIDOSCOPY*

Normal

Evaluate for small
intestinal disease

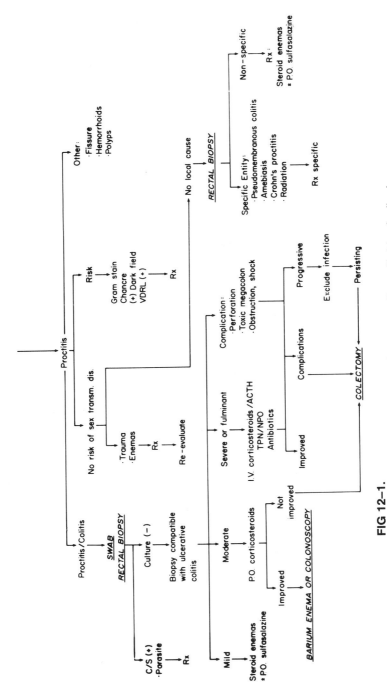

**FIG 12–1.**
Suggested evaluation for the patient presenting with bloody diarrhea.

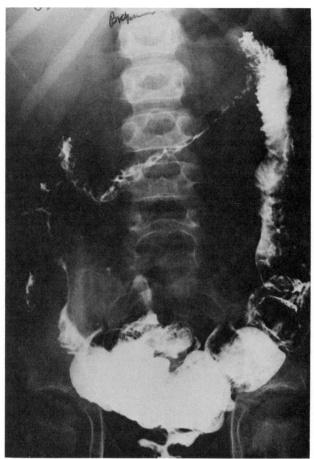

**FIG 12–2.**
Involvement of the terminal ileum, ascending and transverse colon by Crohn's disease. The patient presented with weight loss, crampy abdominal pains, and fever of unknown origin. Note the "string sign" in the terminal ileum. This represents severe narrowing of the lumen due to full thickness involvement, edema, and accompanying spasm. (Courtesy of Walter Berdon, M.D., Director of Pediatric Radiology, Babies Hospital (Presbyterian Hospital), New York.)

As important as judicious use of medications is, a comprehensive approach to the patient is crucial so that the treatment addresses both the physical and the emotional aspects of the illness. At times, the latter become overwhelming. Understanding and support can prevent serious depression and provide needed reassurance and guidance.

Medications can in many cases induce a remission and prolong the interval between exacerbations, but in most cases of Crohn's, the activity of the disease cannot be predicted and steroid dependency can become a distressing handicap.

In the case of ulcerative colitis, it has been shown that prolonged use of sulfasalazine (Azulfidine) is better than placebo in maintaining a remission. Unfortunately, the same is not true for steroids in Crohn's. Nonetheless, in some children who present with growth retardation, accelerated growth can be accomplished with low-dose, alternate-day steroids. A flare-up of the disease during the adolescent spurt can result in serious growth arrest and necessitates another round of everyday high-dose steroids to attempt reinduction of remission.

## Steroids

In the child who presents with growth retardation and has little evidence of activity, a short course of prednisone 1–1.5 mg/kg/day for 2 or 3 weeks can be followed by tapering by 5 mg/day every week until a dose of 15–20 mg/day is reached. At this point, alternate-day tapering can follow, decreasing the dosage by 5 mg/day on alternate days and observing the response for 7–10 days before further decreases. In $1^1/_2$ months, the patient can be on 15 mg to 20 mg every other day. As can be expected, many variations to this regimen have been tried and are used by different practitioners.

It is unusual to develop a cushingoid complexion using this schedule. More commonly, parents report a marked increase in appetite, an improvement in the odor of the stools and in their frequency, and a return to more normal activity and endurance. Patients with active disease will not respond as quickly and will need higher steroids for longer periods. Interestingly, once the disease gets under better control, side effects develop more rapidly, unless the steroids are further tapered.

In ulcerative colitis limited to the rectosigmoid, great symptomatic improvement can often be accomplished by local treatment with *steroid enemas*. Most commonly used preparations contain hydrocortisone (in liquid or foam forms) and are sold in convenient, ready-to-use packages, single-dose or multidose with an applicator. Symptomatic relief or tenesmus occurs in a matter of days. A substantial proportion of the hydrocortisone is absorbed, especially if inflammation is extensive. Adrenal suppression can occur during topical treatment with these preparations.

## Sulfasalazine

Sulfasalazine, introduced for the management of ulcerative colitis 25 years ago, is an interesting compound. It is sulfapyridine (an antibiotic) attached by an azo-bond to 5-aminosalicylic acid (5-ASA), an anti-inflammatory. Until recently it was believed that the antibiotic was responsible for the beneficial effects of the drug, but recent work has documented that it is the aminosalicylate moiety that accounts for the drug's therapeutic effect. The azo-bond is split by bacteria, hence its usefulness in inflammation involving the colon, where the active ingredient can be released. Because most of the allergic side effects are related to the sulfa portion, a derivative containing two 5-ASA molecules attached by an azo-bond is being tested and will become available in the near future.

The most common side effects of sulfasalazine are GI upset and nausea which are improved by taking the medication on a full stomach. Enteric coated preparations have helped solve this problem. The most serious side effects are idiosyncratic reactions ranging from urticaria to severe Stevens-Johnson syndrome. Hepatotoxicity is rare but should be recognized with routine liver function tests in the first weeks of therapy. This is a granulomatous hepatitis, sometimes with features of chronic active disease, believed to be triggered by deposition of immune complexes.

Since sulfasalazine interferes with folate metabolism, a supplement of 1 mg daily or every other day should be routine. Occurrence of skin rashes or signs of liver toxicity are an indication to discontinue sulfasalazine use. Experience with sulfasalazine or 5-ASA enemas has been reported in Europe, mainly for ulcerative colitis, but this preparation has not yet been made available for routine use in the United States.

## Growth Retardation

One of the most common presentations in the young, growth retardation can be often traced to years of deceleration in height velocity. The importance of regular weight and height measurements in children cannot be overemphasized. The adolescent growth spurt is accompanied by a fairly uniform spectrum of development of secondary sex characteristics. Delay in their onset and failure to progress along the guidelines so well described by Tanner are reasons for concern and should not be dismissed as a constitutional trait until proven otherwise.

Awareness of the unusual presentations of inflammatory bowel disease in this age group can make a big difference in the life of the patient. The mistaken diagnosis of anorexia nervosa has devastating effects on the family. A high index of suspicion is needed to rule out an organic source for the symptoms with certainty. Anorexia is indeed common in IBD, and food aversions can resemble an eating disorder, especially if vomiting is a regular occurrence. Delayed menarche or secondary amenorrhea can suggest an endocrine problem. In some patients, the gastrointestinal symptoms are minimal, even after repeated questioning. Perhaps they may recall foul smelling stools or describe a subtle pattern of increased flatus, unformed stools, nausea associated with eating, or abdominal distention. Most of these comments apply to Crohn's disease of the small intestine, since colitis, as a rule, will be more evident due to the common occurrence of bleeding or abnormal stools.

### Etiology of Growth Retardation

The etiology of growth retardation in IBD appears to be mainly related to malnutrition. Studies of protein turnover in children receiving steroids failed to show an effect of inflammation on rate of synthesis or catabolism. Malabsorption can worsen the malnutrition, but even when no measurable steatorrhea is detectable, poor growth can be traced to consumption of insufficient amounts of energy and, to a lesser extent, protein.

The importance of trace minerals in permitting normal adolescent development has focused on zinc, since studies from the Middle East reported the association between delayed growth and this trace mineral deficiency. In certain areas of Egypt and Iran, bread is very rich in fiber and promotes abnormal losses of minerals, including zinc. Hypogonadism and infantilism were also described, and correction with zinc supplements was dramatic. Zinc is an important trace mineral because of its role as a cofactor in such enzymes as DNA synthetase, alkaline phosphatase, lactic dehydrogenase, and scores of others. Increased losses in IBD (also in short bowel syndrome, high ileostomies, cystic fibrosis, and chelation therapy) have been reported.

### Management of Growth Retardation

The route and choice of nutritional supplementation will be dictated by the extent and degree of disease activity, the presence of partial obstruction or fistulas, associated lactase deficiency, steatorrhea from terminal ileal dysfunction, and bile salt depletion or bacterial overgrowth.

In the mildest forms, it is possible to provide additional calories (30%–40% above requirements for height-age) in the form of high calorie drinks or puddings. Many of the commercially available products are lactose-free and usually well tolerated, except for excessive fullness and flavor fatigue. If there is no lactose intolerance, satisfactory replacement for proprietary supplements can be "concocted" with milk, cream, eggs, ice cream, and malts. It is important to determine lactose tolerance before instituting any supplementation program in order to avoid severe exacerbation of diarrhea and cramping.

Ongoing studies suggest a therapeutic role for *elemental diets* in the management of inflammatory bowel disease. Elemental or chemically defined diets contain a mixture of amino acids and a carbohydrate source, usually glucose and glucose polymers; they are practically fat-free except for essential fatty acids. Elemental diets do not stimulate pancreatic and biliary secretions as much, and are, of course, residue-free. Their absorption takes place in the duodenum and upper jejunum, and fecal flow is markedly decreased. A major drawback is their flavor (or lack of a good one) and the frequent need to administer them by NG

TABLE 12–4.
Most Common Indications for Surgery in Inflammatory Bowel Disease

Ulcerative colitis for longer than a decade or if dysplasia is present
Failure to control inflammation with the full range of medical measures:
  Bowel rest
  Intravenous nutrition
  ACTH, steroids
  Antibiotics
  Immunosuppressives
Unacceptable side effects from therapy
Intractable pain
Massive bleeding
Intestinal obstruction unresponsive to conservative management
Toxic megacolon
Intestinal perforation
Intestinal fistula or abscess
Growth retardation in the prepubertal youngster with limited involvement

tube. In addition, their osmolarity is high, and use of full strength solutions (1 or 1.5 calorie/ml) tends initially to result in nausea and diarrhea.

Preliminary results suggest that remission of Crohn's disease can be induced as effectively with an elemental diet as with steroids. However, remission could not be maintained once the formula was discontinued. In patients with extensive and very active disease, central vein alimentation (TPN) has been shown to be a valuable adjunct to medications. If surgery is indicated, correction of protein-calorie malnutrition with TPN decreases morbidity and mortality.

In the motivated prepubertal youngster with growth retardation, excellent results can often be accomplished by supplemental nocturnal NG feedings. Amazingly, passage of the tube becomes routine, and the accelerated linear growth usually provides a powerful positive reinforcement. Therapy needs to be continued for as long as oral intake is insufficient to maintain adequate growth and maturation.

For the preadolescent patient in whom all medical measures fail to bring relief of symptoms, and when, despite intensive nutritional support, growth failure persists, serious consideration of surgical resection becomes a pressing and difficult issue. The ever-present risks of recurrence need to be weighed against chronic illness, depression, recurrent pain, and inability to function at peer level. A disease-free interval can be of crucial importance during the formative years of college and while developing interpersonal relations. The most common indications for surgery are presented in Table 12–4.

# BIBLIOGRAPHY

1. Kirsner JB, Shorter RG: Recent developments in "nonspecific" inflammatory bowel disease. *N Engl J Med* 1982; 306:775–785, 837–848.
2. Kirschner BS, Licsh JR, Kalman SS, et al: Reversal of growth retardation in Crohn's disease with therapy emphasizing oral nutrition restitution. *Gastroenterology* 1982; 80:10.
3. Morin CL, Roulet M, Roy CC, et al: Continuous enteral alimentation in children with Crohn's disease and growth failure. *Gastroenterology* 1980; 79:1205.
4. Kodner IJ, Fry RD: Inflammatory bowel disease. *Ciba Found Symp* 1982; 34:1–32.
5. Kelts EG, Grand RJ: Inflammatory bowel disease in children and adolescents. *Curr Probl Pediatr* 1980; 10(5):1–40.
6. Grand RJ, Homer DR: Approaches to inflammatory bowel disease in childhood and adolescence. *Pediatr Clin North Am* 1975; 22(4):835–850.
7. Whittington PF, Vedain-Barnes H, Bayless TM: Medical management of Crohn's disease in adolescence. *Gastroenterology.* 1977; 72:1330–1344.
8. Fonkalsrud EW, Ament ME, Byrne WJ: Clinical experience with total colectomy and endorectal mucosal resection for inflammatory bowel disease. *Gastroenterology* 1979; 77:156–160.
9. National Foundation for Ileitis and Colitis. Banks PA, Present DH, Steiner P (eds): *The Crohn's Disease and Ulcerative Colitis Fact Book.* New York, Charles Scribner & Sons, 1983.
10. Booth IW, Harries JT: Inflammatory bowel disease in childhood. *Gut* 1984; 25:188–202.
11. Rosenthal SR, Snyder JD, Hendricks KM, et al: Growth failure and inflammatory bowel disease: Approach to treatment of a complicated adolescent problem. *Pediatrics* 1983; 72(4):481–490.

# 13

## Pancreatitis

The diagnosis of pancreatitis is being made with increasing frequency in infancy and childhood. The possibility of pancreatic inflammation needs to be considered in the evaluation of acute and recurrent abdominal pains, abdominal distention, intermittent jaundice, and vomiting.

No age is spared. In the infant and young child, the underlying etiology is more likely to be related to a congenital anomaly of the bile ducts, the pancreatic ducts, or the duodenum (for example, an enteric duplication). In the toddler, the possibility of trauma needs to be ruled out, especially if child abuse is suspected. Most often, a history of blunt trauma is elicited only after much prodding, since the episode is usually forgotten by then. In the adolescent patient, obesity with associated gallbladder disease and alcohol can be important factors. A listing of the causes of pancreatitis is presented in Table 13–1.

### MECHANISMS OF PANCREATIC INFLAMMATION

The mechanisms of intraglandular activation of pancreatic enzymes have not been fully elucidated. In mechanical obstruction, there is increased intraductal pressure with interference of ductular flow. After prozymogens become activated, a chain reaction can take place in the body of the gland. Reflux of bile, either because of a congenital anomaly in the pancreatic and common bile ducts, or

TABLE 13–1.
Etiology of Pancreatitis

Idiopathic (as high as 20%–30% of cases)
Drugs
    Prednisone
    Thiazides
    Tetracycline
    Azathioprine
    Salicylazosulfapyridine (Azulfadine)
    Oral contraceptives
    L-asparaginase
    Valproic acid
    Furosemide
Other Drugs or Toxins
    Alcohol
    Scorpion poison
Trauma
Congenital or Acquired Structural Anomalies
    Choledochal cyst
    Enteric duplications or cysts (gastric, duodenal)
    Pseudocyst
    Tumor
    Cholelithiasis
Infections
    Viral, bacterial
        Mycoplasma pneumonia
        Mumps, rubella, coxsackie, influenza, hepatitis A and B
        Tuberculosis
    Parasitic (causing obstruction of the pancreatic duct)
        Ascaris
        Echinococcus
        Clonorchis sinensis
Metabolic Disorders
    Hyperparathyroidism
    Hyperlipidemia types I, IV, V
    Aminoacidurias
    Vitamin D deficiency
    Hypercalcemia
    Reye's syndrome
Hereditary Conditions
    Cystic fibrosis
    Familial recurrent pancreatitis
Collagen Vascular Disease
    Lupus erythematosus
    Periateritis nodosa

because of back flow secondary to obstruction in the ampulla of Vater, can also be a triggering factor to the activation of digestive enzymes. The mechanisms of damage in metabolic disorders such as the hyperlipidemias or hyperparathyroidism are not fully understood.

## HEMORRHAGIC AND INTERSTITIAL PANCREATITIS

### *Pathology*

Pancreatitis can present suddenly, with inflammation progressing in a matter of hours to complete autolysis of the gland. Hemorrhagic infarction, severe edema, activation of the clotting cascade, and peritonitis will be present in these fulminant cases. Calcifications can occur, with saponification of lipids in the pancreas or other distant locations. Superimposed infection with enteric organisms, abscess or phlegmon formation, and resolution with the development of a pseudocyst can also take place.

In less fulminant cases, exudative inflammation is present. Edema distends the interstitial spaces of the gland; inflammatory cells and fibroblasts accumulate among the acini, but diffuse necrosis does not take place.

### Pain in Pancreatitis

The severity and location of the pain during an attack of pancreatitis can be understood by remembering the anatomical relations to the celiac plexus and its autonomic innervation. The pancreas is a retroperitoneal structure with its sensory innervation being part of the network of sympathetic and vagal efferents shared by other upper abdominal viscera. Thoracic segments T5–9 and T10–11 harbor the preganglionic elements of the efferent loop and, when stimulated, refer their sensation to cutaneous dermatomes supplied by T7–8–9 and to the low thoracic spine. The anatomical relationship between the pancreas and its surrounding structures is presented in Figure 13–1.

Typically, the pain of pancreatic inflammation is upper epigastric in location. Surprisingly, even with severe involvement, accompanying guarding and rebound might not be dramatic. In other instances, peritoneal irritation from released enzymes can be extreme, producing a "board-like" abdomen due to diffuse abdominal wall muscle spasm. The patient tends to avoid all movement and assumes a withdrawn position with hips flexed. If diaphragmatic irritation has occurred, respirations will be shallow, with splinting and grunting.

### Clinical Features

Abdominal pain is the most common presenting symptom, midepigastric in a majority of patients, as mentioned before, but also diffuse, periumbilical, or

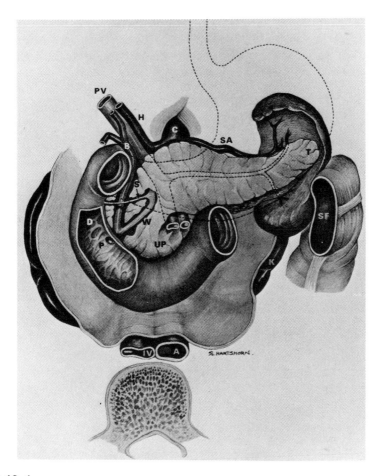

**FIG 13–1.**
Anatomical relationships between the pancreas and its surrounding structures. *A* = abdominal aorta; *IV* = inferior vena cava; *K* = left kidney; *P* = ampulla of Vater; *W* = main pancreatic duct; *D* = duodenum; *T* = tail; *S* = accessory pancreatic duct; *B* = common bile duct; *PV* = portal vein; *C* = celiac trunk; *SF* = splenic flexure, colon. (From Howat HT, Sarles H (eds): *The Exocrine Pancreas.* Philadelphia, WB Saunders Co, 1979. Used by permission.)

radiating to the back. Occasionally, pancreatitis can present with right lower quadrant pain, raising the possibility of acute appendicitis.

Pain is worsened by eating and by movement. Nausea and vomiting are also common, occurring in over 75% of the cases. Temperature elevation can be marked and can last for days or even weeks. Spiking fevers, progressive abdominal rigidity, and toxicity suggest hemorrhagic destruction and are worrisome signs. Paralytic ileus is common, and pleural effusions occur more frequently in adults. For reasons that are not clear, effusions are preferentially located on the left side. Ascites can develop rapidly or may even be the presenting feature in young children.

### Laboratory and Radiologic Examinations

The definitive diagnosis of pancreatitis can only be made by pathological examination of the organ. Unfortunately, in fulminant cases, the patient will come to autopsy. Unsuspected pancreatitis can occasionally be discovered incidentally. Serum amylase activity greater than three times the established normal level is usually strongly suggestive of pancreatitis. Amylase activity increases as a function of age, from a low of less than 30 Somogyi units at birth to about 90 units in adolescence.

Problems with interpretation of serum amylase levels stem from the nonspecific elevation seen in cases of biliary tract disease, intestinal inflammation, or perforating peptic ulcer. On the other hand, cases of proven pancreatitis can present with normal serum amylase. Because amylase is readily filtered by the kidney, the elevation in the serum can be brief (hours to days) and be missed completely.

Measuring the *amylase clearance* in the urine and expressing it as the ratio to creatinine clearance has been found to be more sensitive and more specific than isolated serum amylase determinations, at least in adults.

The ratio of the clearances is calculated by simultaneously measuring serum amylase and creatinine, and urine amylase and creatinine. A 24-urine collection is not needed:

$$Ac/Cc = Sa \times Sc/Uc \times Ua \times 100$$

*where*

$Ac$ = amylase clearance
$Cc$ = creatinine clearance
$Sa$ = serum amylase
$Sc$ = serum creatinine
$Uc$ = urine creatinine
$Ua$ = urine analysis

The ratio, expressed as a percent, is below 4% in normal individuals and rises to over 10% in acute pancreatitis. In hyperamylasemia due to causes other than pancreatitis, this ratio does not increase. Unfortunately, no similar experience has yet been recorded in the pediatric patient. In fact, a study of 13 patients with pancreatitis failed to confirm the reliability of the amylase/creatinine clearance ratio in this population.

From that study and others, it is suggested that abdominal ultrasonography is a more reliable way of detecting pancreatic edema. The echogenicity of the pancreas is almost identical to that of the left lobe of the liver. This comparison can be made reliably by an experienced sonographer. Decreased echogenicity is seen with engorgement and edema of the gland, and development of a pseudocyst or an abscess can be followed closely. This kind of information is crucial to help the clinician decide whether surgical intervention is necessary or to follow the spontaneous resorption of a pseudocyst. Anatomical definition, often crucial to the surgeon, is best accomplished with endoscopic retrograde choledocho-pancreatography (ERCP), which is feasible even in young children. Timing of the procedure is important since flare-up of pancreatitis and bacteremia can follow injection of contrast material in the duct system.

Serum lipase has also been used for the diagnosis of acute pancreatitis since it is cleared from the circulation much slower and therefore remains elevated for a longer time. It is also more specific for pancreatic injury than amylase. The assay is available in most centers.

**Treatment**

The mainstays of therapy remain:

1. Aggressive fluid and electrolyte replacement, including blood and plasma fractions in the fulminant cases.
2. Pain control.
3. Complete reduction of stimulation to the pancreas.

Maintaining the patient *NPO* and providing *nasogastric suction* will diminish the pain in many cases, but not in all. Intractable pain can be distressing, both to the patient and to the doctors attempting to offer relief. Morphine should not be used because of its spasmodic effect on the biliary tree and the sphincter of Oddi, but meperidine has been shown to be well tolerated and should be used in adequate doses, intravenously if necessary. The *H-2 histamine antagonists* (cimetidine, ranitidine, and famotidine) can effectively suppress gastric acid production, further diminishing pancreatic stimulation. The usefulness of anti-cholinergic drugs and prophylactic antibiotic has not been convincingly demonstrated.

In fulminant cases, removal of toxic substances and ascitic fluid by *peritoneal lavage* has been shown to offer a chance to an otherwise desperately ill patient. A controlled study in adults could not confirm the usefulness of this modality of treatment. *Surgical debridement* of the pancreas, evacuation of abscess ma-terial, and necrotic tissue can be lifesaving in those extreme situations.

Careful monitoring is mandatory when pancreatitis is severe. Metabolic derangements involve every important organ and system. Intensive supportive care can see the patient through the crucial acute period. Pulmonary support, control of hypotension, shock maintenance of glucose, calcium homeostasis, and nutritional support are some of the complex therapeutic issues involved in the management of the patient with acute pancreatitis.

After the initial attack subsides, usually within 4 to 10 days, nasogastric suction is discontinued and the patient is observed for abdominal distention, recurrence of nausea, vomiting, or pain. Oral feedings are started cautiously, initially with clear fluids containing carbohydrates. Protein and fat are introduced as tolerated. If a flare-up of pancreatic inflammation occurs, or if there is a marked change in serum amylase activity or urine clearance, feedings should be discontinued and intravenous nutrition provided either by peripheral vein or by central venous line. Further attempts at oral feedings should be deferred until the clinical condition stabilizes and laboratory values show steady improvement.

Deterioration in the patient's condition, abdominal distention, fever, or jaundice suggest the development of a pancreatic pseudocyst, retroperitoneal collection, ascites, or an abscess. Ultrasonographic surveillance is most useful in this respect.

### Chronic Recurrent Pancreatitis

Whether a familial autosomal dominant condition, a consequence of underlying metabolic abnormality (hypercalcemia, hyperlipidemia, etc.), or from anatomical defects, repeated bouts of pancreatitis can result in fibrosis and destruction of the pancreas with serious nutritional consequences. Both exocrine and endocrine function are ultimately affected, and patients require life-long enzyme replacement and insulin for diabetes control. Drug addiction is hard to avoid and morbidity is significant.

## BIBLIOGRAPHY

1. Aldrete J, Jimenez H, Halpern N: Evaluation and treatment of acute and chronic pancreatitis. A review of 380 cases. *Ann Surg* 1980; 191:664.
2. Balart LA, Ferrante WA: Pathophysiology of acute and chronic pancreatitis. *Ann Intern Med* 1982; 142:113.
3. Cox KL, Ament ME, Sample WY, et al: Ultrasonic and biochemical diagnosis of pancreatitis. *J Pediatr* 1980; 96:407.
4. Jordan SC, Ament ME: Pancreatitis in children and adolescents. *J Pediatr* 1977; 91:211.
5. Lebenthal E, Schwachman H: The pancreas—development, adaptation, and malfunction in infancy and childhood. *Clin Gastroenterol* 1977; 6:397.
6. Hillemeier C, Gryboski JD: Acute pancreatitis in infants and children. *Yale J Biol Med* 1984; 57:149–159.
7. Butain WL: Chronic relapsing pancreatitis in childhood. *Am Surg* 1985; 51:180–188.

8. Tam PKH, Saing H, Irving IM, et al: Acute pancreatitis in children. *J Pediatr Surg* 1985; 20:58–60.

9. Ghishan FK, Greene HL, Avant G, et al: Chronic relapsing pancreatitis in childhood. *J Pediatr* 1983; 102:514–518.

10. Neiderau C, Grendell JH: Diagnosis of chronic pancreatitis. *Gastroenterology* 1985; 88:1953–1955.

# 14

## Diseases of the Liver

Recognition of liver dysfunction requires both a high index of suspicion and a thorough physical examination. Symptoms of liver disease can be totally non-specific or draw immediate attention to that organ, either because of abdominal distention, localized pain, or the appearance of jaundice.

In broad terms, the liver can be involved in a number of ways:

- Parenchymal infections (viral, bacterial, mycotic, parasitic)
- Toxic damage, both cholestatic and hepatocellular
- Kupffer cell hyperplasia as a systemic response to infection
- Infiltration with abnormal metabolites (storage diseases): fat, glycogen, etc.
- Infiltration by tumors (primary or secondary)
- Congenital defects resulting in fibrosis or cystic changes
- Engorgement by impaired blood flow such as occurs in congestive heart failure or hepatic vein obstruction (Budd-Chiari syndrome).

Symptoms of liver disease can be subtle, and most cases of infectious hepatitis are asymptomatic. Among the most common signs and symptoms to look for and recognize are:

*Signs*
    1. Abdominal distention
       a. Hepatomegaly

    b. Splenomegaly
    c. Ascites
    d. Masses
  2. Jaundice, bronze- or green-colored skin
  3. Dark urine
  4. Light colored stools, steatorrhea
  5. Xanthoma
  6. Spider angiomata
  7. Liver palms and soles
  8. Clubbing of nails
  9. Short stature
 10. Ecchymoses, bleeding diathesis.

*Symptoms*

  1. Localized tenderness in right upper quadrant, shoulder
  2. Tiredness
  3. Malaise
  4. Fever
  5. Nausea, vomiting
  6. Anorexia, weight loss
  7. Itching
  8. Mental changes, insomnia, irritability.

With the introduction and widespread use of biochemical screen tests, abnormal liver function is being encountered unexpectedly. In this way, slight elevation of the total bilirubin or transaminases are being detected, promoting further investigations and repeat blood work to confirm or rule out the abnormalities. Most cases of *Gilbert's syndrome* are recognized incidentally. It has also become apparent that the liver can be involved during intercurrent viral infections such as varicella or Coxsackie. In addition, medications taken for acute or chronic conditions can affect the level of the transaminases or induce a mild cholestatic reaction. Aspirin, erythromycin, and antineoplastic drugs are but a few of the long list of potential offenders. A more complete listing is provided (Table 14–1).

## Assessment of Liver Dysfunction

Included among the "liver function tests" are measurements of different sensitivity and specificity. Most commonly used tests are really not a measure of liver function but rather *static measures* reflecting leakage of enzymes from the hepatocyte and biliary epithelium, membrane, cytosol, or organelles.

More specific and *dynamic tests* include the *aminopyrine breath test, ga-*

TABLE 14–1.

Hepatotoxic Agents (Partial Listing)

ANESTHETICS
  Carbon tetrachloride
  Enflurane
  Halothane
ANALGESICS
  Acetaminophen
  Phenylbutazone
  Sulindac
ANTICONVULSANTS AND TRANQUILIZERS
  Phenytoin
  Valproate
  Carbamazepine
  Phenobarbital
  Phenothiazines
  Chlordiazepoxide
  Haloperidol
  Diazepam
ANTIBIOTICS
  Arsenicals
  Erythromycin
  Isoniazid
  Rifamycin
  Sulfonamides
  Nitrofurantoin
  Tetracycline
CARDIOVASCULAR
  Methyldopa
  Procainamide
  Quinidine
  Clofibrate
IMMUNOSUPPRESSANTS
  Methotrexate
  L-asparaginase
  6-Mercaptopurine
  Azathioprine
  Puromycin

*lactose* and *bile acid clearances*, or *dye excretions*, most of which are not routinely used in clinical practice. These tests are much better indicators of total hepatic cell mass and reflect the liver's metabolic and excretory capacities. Recently, the elimination of caffeine in saliva has been found to be a promising and simple method of determining hepatic functional reserve.

Caution is always indicated when interpreting results. A good test is one that not only detects patients with liver disease and excludes those without it (high sensitivity) but is able to detect those who do not have liver disease (high specificity). The use of a whole battery of tests when assessing liver dysfunction improves the sensitivity and specificity of the evaluation.

The serum SGOT, LDH, and the alkaline phosphatase are three commonly, if insensitive, static indicators of liver function. The SGOT, or better named AST (aspartate aminotransferase), is found also in red cells and muscle and can be elevated in hemolysis, whether it happens in vivo or in vitro, after blood drawing. The same is true for LDH (lactic dehydrogenase), an enzyme found in red cells, white cells, and lung, among other tissues. The alkaline phosphatase is normally elevated in growing children and adolescents, sometimes in the 200 IU range. Obstruction to bile flow results in increased production of this enzyme and subsequent backflow into the plasma. Alkaline phosphatase is also present in the small intestine, certain tumors, and in the placenta.

A more specific way to detect biliary disease is measuring the activity of gamma glutamyl transpeptidase (GGTP), found in the bile duct epithelium and liver cells and not affected by bone growth. The 5′ nucleotidase was popular for a while as a marker of cholestasis; the GGTP has proven to be more reliable.

Another important marker of cholestasis is the cholesterol concentration. As a result of prolonged impairment to bile flow, cholesterol concentration rises, sometimes to extremely high levels, sufficient to cause its deposition in the skin as xanthomata. The SGPT, or better called alanine aminotransferase (ALT), is more specific than the SGOT since it is not bound to organelles in the hepatocyte and its appearance in the circulation reflects liver cell damage.

## Synthetic Function Tests

Measures of the liver's synthetic capacities are the albumin concentration and the clotting factors, as measured by various coagulation tests. Albumin has a half life of 12 days and therefore will not decrease immediately. The liver has the capacity to double albumin synthesis in the face of increased losses (renal, intestinal). It is a good measure of overall synthetic function, and its declining concentration (without associated losses) correlates with prognosis in liver failure.

The vitamin K dependent factors, II, VII, and IX, are primarily measured by the quick prothrombin time (PT). The partial thromboplastin time (APTT) is also prolonged in liver disease. When abnormally prolonged PT and APTT fail to correct after administration of parenteral vitamin K, serious and sometimes irreversible deterioration of liver function is present.

Abnormalities in fibrinogen function have been described and can result in abnormal tests without actual coagulopathy. When a low fibrinogen concentration is measured in liver disease, diffuse intravascular coagulation needs always to be considered, but the possibility of dysfibrinogenemia should be kept in mind. This can be documented by measuring fibrinogen concentrations directly, with a radioimmunoassay.

**Liver Imaging**

Accurate anatomic identification of some causes of liver disease is now possible with use of ultrasound, computerized tomography, and isotope scanning. In addition, the possibility of visualizing the biliary tree by percutaneous injection of contrast material (transhepatic cholangiography) has become a reality even for young children and infants. Flexible needles (Chiba, "skinny" needles) make the liver puncture innocuous under adequate anesthesia and immobility, and have become very useful in the investigation of bile duct abnormalities such as sclerosing cholangitis or cystic dilatations.

Ultrasonography (especially real-time) is, in experienced hands, the modality of choice for the initial investigation of conjugated hyperbilirubinemia. In a noninvasive way, it can immediately detect bile duct dilatation, identify the gallbladder, image gallstones, ascites, and space-occupying lesions. Spleen size can be measured. Doppler ultrasound can be used for identification of blood flow in the presence of portal hypertension and associated increased collateral circulation.

Isotopes injected in the circulation and extracted by the reticuloendothelial system are useful in delineating liver and spleen sizes, focal abnormalities, and overall hepatocyte function.

Technetium (Tc) 99m has a half-life of 6 hours and is a weak gamma radiation emitter. Sulfur colloid labelled with technetium 99m is widely used for investigation of hepatosplenomegaly. Shift of the isotope to the kidneys and bone marrow is an additional indication of hepatic cell dysfunction.

To visualize the biliary system, the family of imidodiacetic (IDA) compounds is now used, completely replacing the [131]I-rose bengal test. Also labelled with technetium 99m, this isotope is handled as bilirubin and other anionic dyes. After conjugation in the liver cells, it is excreted via the bile canaliculi and bile ducts. Visualization of the gallbladder is not always possible, but detecting the presence of isotope in the intestine is positive proof of a patent bile duct system (provided no abnormal fistula exist). Unfortunately, in the presence of severe cholestasis and hepatocellular disease, retention of the tracer in the liver can be complete, simulating bile duct obstruction.

**Liver Biopsy**

Liver biopsy is indicated in cases of undiagnosed cholestatic jaundice, especially in the neonatal period when the distinction between extrahepatic biliary atresia and neonatal hepatitis is so crucial for adequate management.

The significance of persistently abnormal liver function tests can at times be assessed only by direct examination of liver tissue. Distinction between chronic active and chronic persistent hepatitis is made on morphologic grounds, and consideration of treatment with steroids in the former and watchful waiting in the second is only possible with this information.

Identification of the cause of hepatomegaly (storage disorders, fat, glycogen, tumor, hepatitis, etc.) is also possible with enzymatic determinations for certain inborn errors of metabolism in tissue obtained by percutaneous biopsy.

Major contraindications for a percutaneous biopsy include:

- Ascites (the liver tends to float away, risking leaks and perforation to other viscera)
- Suspected vascular lesion (hemangiomas, etc.)
- Coagulation abnormalities, thrombocytopenia
- Pleural effusions, especially if infected, when a subcostal approach is not possible
- Liver abscesses or other cystic lesions (i.e., echinococcus)
- Unruly patient.

When performed with proper preparation by an experienced gastroenterologist or surgeon, the technique has a low rate of serious complications (less than 0.6%) and plays a definite and important role in the diagnosis and management of liver disorders.

## BIBLIOGRAPHY

1. Carlisle R, Galambos JT, Warren D: The relationship between conventional liver tests, quantitative function tests, and histopathology in cirrhosis. *Dig Dis Sci* 1979; 24:358–362.
2. Jost G, Wahllander A, Mandach U et al: Overnight salivary caffeine clearance: A liver function test suitable for routine use. *Hepatology* 1987; 7:338–344.

# 15

## Jaundice

Discoloration of the skin and sclera by bilirubin is an important clinical finding that should always be accounted for. If the yellowish discoloration is not present in the sclera and appears more prominent on the palms and soles (especially in children of fair complexion), the first distinction that needs to be made is whether the color is due to carotene pigments rather than bilirubin, since carotenemia is a totally benign condition.

In assessing the infant with jaundice, it is helpful to remember the metabolism and fate of bilirubin, the mechanisms of elevation, and the differential diagnosis of conditions associated with hyperbilirubinemia in the various age groups. Much information has become available in the past 10 years about bilirubin transport into the hepatocyte and its conjugation and secretion into the bile canaliculus. The process will be presented briefly, and the reader is encouraged to amplify this information with the references provided at the end of the chapter. The sophistication reached in the past few years in the description of molecular events at the level of the plasma and the canalicular membranes is truly remarkable and has already begun to find practical applications in the diagnosis and management of cholestatic conditions.

### ORIGIN AND FATE OF BILIRUBIN

Bilirubin is an orange pigment derived from the heme nucleus of hemoglobin. Ninety percent of the bilirubin produced in humans is formed in the spleen and

148

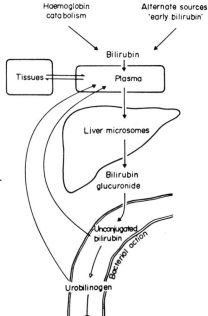

Haemoglobin
catabolism

Alternate sources
'early bilirubin'

Bilirubin

Tissues — Plasma

Liver microsomes

Bilirubin
glucuronide

Unconjugated
bilirubin

Bacterial action

Urobilinogen

**FIG 15–1.**
Schematic representation of the pathways of bilirubin metabolism. (From Sherlock S: *Diseases of the Liver and the Biliary System*, ed 6. Boston, Blackwell Scientific Publications, 1981. Used by permission.)

the liver from hemoglobin metabolism after effete, red cells are removed by the reticuloendothelial system (Fig 15–1). Some bilirubin is produced in the bone marrow from inefficient synthesis of hemoglobin during erythropoiesis ("shunt" bilirubinemia). Metabolism of nonheme proteins, such as cytochrome C or myoglobin, accounts for less than 5% of total bilirubin production.

The first metabolite in the conversion of heme into bilirubin is biliverdin, a reaction that is enzymatically controlled by the enzyme heme oxygenase located in the microsomes. This step is rate limiting and generates carbon monoxide and biliverdin which in turn is degraded to bilirubin by the ubiquitous enzyme bilirubin reductase. For transport from the site of production to the liver, bilirubin is bound to albumin tightly. Drugs administered to the infant can compete for the same binding sites displacing the bilirubin and enhancing its toxicity.

This water-insoluble bilirubin is measured by the routine diazo reaction as the "indirect fraction." The Van de Bergh reaction is still the most commonly performed fractionation technique, and despite its limitations, it seems to provide a useful screening method to separate bilirubin into its water-soluble (direct) and water-insoluble (indirect) components.

The deleterious effects of bilirubin to the infant's brain are entirely due to the indirect fraction. Because of its fat solubility, it can cross the blood brain barrier and interact with the central nervous system resulting in the clinical syndrome of kernicterus.

## UPTAKE AND CONJUGATION

Through a process not completely understood, the bilirubin-albumin complex dissociates, the bilirubin is brought into the hepatocyte, and is then further metabolized in the endoplasmic reticulum. It is clear that receptors on the membrane are responsible for the transport into the cell of many anions (including bilirubin) and many other molecular species including dyes, fatty acids, lipoproteins, dimeric IgA, etc. Other proteins have been described that are responsible for the binding and transport of bilirubin from the cell membrane to the intracellular organelles involved in its metabolism. Ligandin and Z protein are two of the most likely candidates in this process of facilitated diffusion into the hepatocyte.

Bilirubin is then glucuronidated in a process that requires energy, glucose, uridine, and the presence of the enzyme uridine diphosphoglucuronyl transferase (UDPG-transferase). Conjugation probably involves several steps and generates both monoglucuronides and diglucuronides. Distribution and concentration of these conjugates is being studied for the differentiation of hyperbilirubinemic syndromes such as Gilbert's, Rotor, and Dubin-Johnson. At this time, such distinctions can be only made by application of methodology not available in most clinical laboratories; it remains a research tool waiting for more widespread applications.

## EXCRETION

Following conjugation, bilirubin is transferred to the bile canaliculus where it joins the other components of bile (water, electrolytes, bile acids, phospholipids, cholesterol, and lecithin) and is directed to the gallbladder through the common hepatic and cystic ducts. There it undergoes concentration until the neurohormonal stimuli discharge it—via the common bile duct—into the small intestine. In the large intestine, bilirubin conjugates are further metabolized by colonic bacteria.

Only conjugated bilirubin can be filtered by the kidney and appear in the urine. This occurs in any condition of impaired bile flow whether due to damaged hepatocytes or to obstruction of the bile ducts. On the other hand, the urine will be negative for bilirubin whenever the underlying hyperbilirubinemia is of the indirect type. Sensitive urine dipstick tests are available for the detection of bile pigments and can provide useful information at the bedside early in the workup of the patient with jaundice.

## APPROACH TO THE JAUNDICED PATIENT

Because of the basic differences in the mechanism of production of conjugated and unconjugated hyperbilirubinemia, it is of utmost importance to make that distinction early. As mentioned before, indirect hyperbilirubinemia is dangerous only when the levels are excessive during the newborn period. A moderate increase during the first week or two of life is indeed considered "physiologic" (see below).

In contrast, *direct hyperbilirubinemia is never physiologic* and requires investigation to explain its origin. It is possible to occasionally observe slight increases in the direct fraction when severe hemolysis is present, but this is the exception rather than the rule. The workup of direct hyperbilirubinemia should be approached systematically to promptly rule out the more serious cases and avoid temporizing explanations that only delay proper evaluation and diagnosis.

## INDIRECT (UNCONJUGATED) HYPERBILIRUBINEMIA

Remembering the pathway from heme to bilirubin transport and conjugation in the hepatocyte, the most important mechanisms for the production of an elevated indirect fraction of the serum bilirubin include:

1. Increased red cell turnover and overproduction from increased heme metabolism:
    a. Blood group incompatibility (ABO, Rh, other)
    b. Red cell enzymopathies (spherocytic and nonspherocytic hemolytic anemias, i.e., glucose-6-PD, etc.)
    c. Polycythemia (delayed clamping of the cord, twin-to-twin transfusion)
    d. Extravasated blood (hematomas at various locations)
2. Impaired bilirubin uptake and conjugation
    a. Immaturity of uptake systems
    b. Competition by circulating drugs or bacterial toxins, free fatty acids
    c. Effect of hypoxia, hypoglycemia, acidosis, dehydration, hypothyroidism
    d. Absent UDPG transferase
        • Complete absence: Crigler-Najjar Arias Type I
        • Partial absence: Crigler-Najjar Arias Type II
    e. Mixed etiology: Gilbert's syndrome
3. Increased intestinal reabsorption of bilirubin
    a. Delayed passage of meconium
    b. Pyloric stenosis or high intestinal obstruction
    c. Dehydration.

## PHYSIOLOGIC JAUNDICE

Physiologic jaundice is a common occurrence and is seen in over 70% of otherwise healthy infants. It should appear after the first day of life, and in the full-term infant, it should not rise above 6–7 mg% at its peak on the third or fourth day of life, with clearance within one week. The limits are different for the premature infant where values of 12 to 15 mg% are acceptable and where return to normal can be delayed for two full weeks.

Jaundice appearing in the first 4 hours after birth or present at birth is *not* physiologic, and another explanation should be sought to account for it. In most cases, a hemolytic process is responsible for early jaundice and requires close monitoring to prepare for exchange transfusion if the rate of increase exceeds the accepted limits.

The mechanism of physiologic jaundice remains an unsettled issue, although it appears to be the result of factors producing increased bilirubin synthesis from increased red cell turnover, decreased uptake at the level of the hepatocyte, and probably increased enterohepatic circulation of bilirubin.

The role of the physician in charge of the care of the neonate is to screen promptly for conditions leading to abnormal levels of hyperbilirubinemia and to institute exchange transfusion or phototherapy as necessary.

## PHOTOTHERAPY

Exposure to visible radiation in the range of 400–500 nm with radiation fluxes of 4–6 $\mu W/m^2/min$ has proven very useful in preventing too rapid a rise in the unconjugated fraction of bilirubin and has spared many infants from exchange transfusion. Light at this wavelength excites the bilirubin molecule and produces various photoisomers, which are unstable and further degrade into compounds cleared via the urine and also via the hepatocyte without need for conjugation. In contrast, exposing conjugated bilirubin to light tends to favor the formation of degradation products which give the skin a greenish discoloration, very typical of infants with cholestatic jaundice, and quite different from the yellowish tint seen in infants with indirect hyperbilirubinemia.

Interesting reports have appeared on the association of phototherapy with loose stools, but the mechanism remains undefined. It is possible that some of the degradation metabolites that are then excreted through the bile into the intestine can be responsible for stimulation of intestinal secretion. A direct effect on the brush border, with interference in the normal function of lactase or other enzymes, could produce lactose intolerance and osmotic diarrhea.

Care should be taken in avoiding dehydration in the infant receiving phototherapy, since insensible water losses are estimated to increase by 20%–30%, and dehydration can worsen the extent and duration of the hyperbilirubinemia. Damage to the retina has also been reported in infants where proper shielding of the eyes was not enforced.

The usefulness of phototherapy is not only limited to the infant in the nursery, but has been extended to the patient with Crigler-Najjar type I, in whom it may be the only practical way to prevent excessive elevations of the bilirubin.

## CRIGLER-NAJJAR SYNDROME

In the infant without a hematological explanation for rapid, severe, indirect hyperbilirubinemia (i.e., blood group or Rh incompatibility, enzymopathy), the diagnosis of Crigler-Najjar should be considered early and an attempt be made to differentiate between type I and type II on the basis of the response to phenobarbital. In type I there is a complete and permanent absence of the conjugating enzyme UDP glucuronyl transferase, while in the type II variant, the enzyme is functionally deficient but not totally; therefore, bilirubin elevations are never very high, in the range below 20 mg%. Kernicterus is unusual.

Type I presents soon after birth, the bilirubin levels reach 40 mg% and more, and the patients will frequently develop kernicterus. The diagnosis can be confirmed by measurement of the activity of UDP glucuronyl transferase in a liver biopsy specimen.

## GILBERT'S SYNDROME

This diagnosis is very rarely made in the neonatal period. Most commonly, mild jaundice might be detected in a youngster or adult during a routine blood multichannel screen, or during an intercurrent illness. The increase in the bilirubin levels is in the range of 2 to 6 mg% and is all unconjugated. It is important to document normal transaminases and to look for occult hemolysis. Unfortunately, there is no routine test that will help make a positive diagnosis, although, as previously mentioned, identification of mono- and diglucuronide conjugates in serum might become a more reliable test in the future. The jaundice tends to increase after fasting or ingesting a diet low in fat. Patients might notice an association between the bilirubin elevations and ill-defined complaints such as lassitude, malaise, nausea, and occasionally, abdominal pains, usually epigastric.

It remains a diagnosis of exclusion, but it is important to reassure the patient of the benign nature of the disorder. Physical activity does not have to be curtailed, and the patient should be informed of the nature of the abnormality so that erroneous and more serious diagnoses are not entertained if the bilirubin elevation is detected during an intercurrent illness.

## BREAST MILK JAUNDICE

A small number of breast-fed infants will develop unconjugated bilirubinemia during the first 2 weeks of life. The bilirubin concentrations can reach levels as high as 15–20 mg%. If breast feedings are continued, the levels tend to fall progressively over the ensuing 4 months. There is no evidence of hemolysis or any other cause for the jaundice and the infants are otherwise healthy and thriving.

Initial observations 20 years ago suggested the presence of an *abnormal steroid* derived from progesterone (pregnane-3-alpha, 20-beta-diol) in the breast milk which competitively inhibited glucuronyl transferase. Those observations could not be duplicated in more recent attempts, so the exact role of pregnanediol in this syndrome remains unsettled.

*Free fatty* acids are produced by the action of lipoprotein lipase on breast milk triglycerides. Evidence suggests that breast milks rich in this enzyme are also more inhibitory of glucuronide transferase activity (especially if linoleic acid concentrations are elevated). This effect can be prevented by boiling the milk, but not by deep freezing at −20°C. The mechanism of action of free fatty acid-mediated hyperbilirubinemia has not yet been fully explained.

Another suspected factor contributing to jaundice in some breast-fed infants is *increased bilirubin reabsorption* somehow promoted by the abnormal milk. Increased enterohepatic recirculation of bilirubin might overload an immature conjugating system.

### Management

Contrary to common belief, supplementation of breast feedings with glucose water (but not plain water) tends to produce *higher* bilirubin concentrations in breast-fed infants when measured during the first 3 days of life. It is also likely that caloric restriction during those days might contribute to the hyperbilirubinemia, similar to the situation in Gilbert's syndrome, or perhaps through increased bilirubin reabsorption from the intestine as has been shown to occur during starvation.

Frequent breast feedings (every 2 hours, for example) and no sugar water supplements can decrease the incidence of prolonged hyperbilirubinemia in the breast-fed infant. If the bilirubin concentrations remain below 20 mg% in the full-term infant, there is no reason to be overly concerned or to discontinue nursing. Experience suggests that a brief interruption of nursing (3 to 4 days), during which time a proprietary formula is given instead, can bring a quicker resolution of breast-milk jaundice even if breast feedings are exclusively resumed after this period.

# CONJUGATED HYPERBILIRUBINEMIA

The finding of an elevated conjugated bilirubin requires prompt evaluation to rule out liver or bile duct pathology. If this fractionation is carried routinely in any infant whose jaundice persists beyond 1 or 2 weeks (for the full-term and premature infant, respectively), early identification of a group of children who need corrective surgery for atresia of the extrahepatic bile ducts is possible, with improved prognosis. In addition, recognition of metabolic abnormalities prevents progressive deterioration if the right dietary changes are instituted. Some conditions will be intractable, and the main contribution with proper diagnosis is in providing genetic counseling to the family.

*Mechanisms*

Conjugated hyperbilirubinemia results from (1) factors affecting hepatocyte function once bilirubin has been transported into the cell, (2) on its way to the bile canaliculus, or (3) from abnormalities in the biliary system, both functional and anatomical.

*Pathological Features*

Interestingly, the liver of the infant shows a limited range of histological changes when subjected to a multitude of injurious stimuli, whether chemical or infectious. The formation of ballooned, *giant cells* is a frequent occurrence in the various neonatal hepatitis syndromes, regardless of their etiology. *Cholestasis*, both intracellular and canalicular, is prominent, and *inflammatory cells* can be seen scattered around the portal tracts and among the hepatocytes.

Several features can be of great help in the differential diagnosis, particularly the presence of bile duct proliferation and intrahepatic granules which stain positively with para-amino-salicylate (PAS) and resist digestion with a diastase. *Bile duct proliferation* is a common response seen in prolonged extrahepatic obstruction, while positive *PAS-diastase resistant granules* are strongly suggestive of alpha-1-antitrypsin deficiency. Expansion of the portal tracts, increased *fibrosis*, collapse of the normal architecture, and *bridging necrosis* can be seen in the liver biopsy.

The final result of progressive liver damage in chronic cholestasis is *biliary cirrhosis*, characterized by increased deposition of collagen from portal tract to portal tract, diffuse obliteration of the medium- and large-sized bile canaliculi, and compression of the portal vasculature by encroaching fibrosis. This results in diversion of portal vein flow, portal hypertension, and its consequences as described in Chapter 18.

## APPROACH TO THE PATIENT WITH CONJUGATED JAUNDICE

Once it has been determined that the elevated bilirubin is conjugated, a systematic approach will help expedite the workup, which should optimally be carried out in a facility where laboratories are available for reliable serodiagnosis, bacteriological and metabolic studies, and experienced imaging radiology. A careful history and physical examination can provide important clues, which help narrow the wide range of possibilities during the initial assessment.

The four major categories of problems to be considered in the differential diagnosis include infectious, metabolic, anatomic, and familial.

### Infections

The presence of prematurity, microcephaly, intracranial calcifications, seizures, and retinitis suggest a congenital viral infection. Involvement of other systems (myocarditis, pneumonia, skin rashes, splenomegaly, thrombocytopenia) also points to a diffuse infectious process.

The most common viruses causing hepatitis in the neonatal period include:

- Cytomegalovirus
- Rubella
- Herpes simplex
- Coxsackie B
- Hepatitis B.

Less frequently seen are:

- Varicella-Zoster
- Echovirus
- Adenovirus.

Occasionally a virus or evidence of viral infection (rubella, cytomegalovirus) can be found in patients who eventually turn out to have complete atresia of the extrahepatic ducts, and therefore a positive demonstration of patent bile ducts is imperative to prevent unnecessary delays in corrective surgery.

Bacterial infections can produce cholestasis by mechanisms not entirely clear, although endotoxin has been implicated. The presence of a urinary tract infection or septicemia should be ruled out by appropriate tests since in many cases, clinical signs are meager. The jaundice will clear after the infection is eradicated with adequate antibiotic therapy. Serologic tests for syphilis and toxoplasmosis drawn in the mother and infant simultaneously will help identify those patients who require specific treatment. When available, specific IgM antibodies will support the diagnosis of an active infection. An elevated total IgM concentration is also suggestive of an intrauterine infection and should be included in the workup of the infant with neonatal jaundice.

## Metabolic

Inborn errors in the metabolism of galactose and fructose can produce severe and irreversible damage to the liver. Accumulation of intermediary metabolites account for the hepatotoxicity, but the exact mechanism of injury has not been determined.

## Galactosemia

Galactosemia should be ruled out in any infant with conjugated jaundice who presents with feeding difficulties, lethargy, or seizures. The deficiency of galactose-1-phosphate-uridyl transferase causes accumulation of galactose-1-phosphate, a hepatotoxin. In addition, this should inhibit the hydrolysis of glycogen, resulting in hypoglycemia and CNS damage. The presence of reducing substances in the urine can be easily tested by the Benedict reaction (Clinitest). If the same specimen is negative for glucose (Testape, or other methods based on the specific glucose oxidase reaction) while the infant is receiving lactose in the diet, galactosemia is a definite diagnostic possibility. It is important to perform the tests while the patient is receiving lactose. Definitive diagnosis is made by direct measurement of the enzyme activity in red blood cells.

If the diagnosis is delayed and lactose intake continues, fatty infiltration progresses to frank cirrhosis, sometimes in a fulminant manner, with splenomegaly, coagulopathy, and ascites in the first few weeks of life.

Galactosemia is not common, occurring in an estimated 1 in 50,000 births.

## Hereditary Fructose Intolerance

Also a rare disease, fructose intolerance can present in infancy if sucrose or fructose is added to the diet, usually as table sugar or honey in drinking water or as a sweetener to cereals and fruits. Sucrose-containing formulas also are available (more frequently in Europe), and an inquiry should always be made as to the specific ingredients and composition of the diet.

The defect involves the activity of the enzyme 1-phosphofructoaldolase, with resulting inability to metabolize fructose-1-phosphate, which can then accumulate in the liver. Inhibition of glycogen hydrolysis also occurs in this condition and results in hypoglycemia, which can often be severe and life threatening. Abnormal activity of a second enzyme, 1,6-diphosphofructoaldolase and accumulation of the diphosphated fructose seems to play a role in causing liver damage and may not return to a normal levels even after instituting a strict fructose-free diet.

The prognosis is not always good, due to the complexity of the metabolic pathways affected and the various mechanisms of liver involvement. There is genetic variability in the expression of this disorder, and progressive liver disease can result in early cirrhosis and liver failure.

A fructose tolerance test should be done with extreme caution because of the serious risk of profound hypoglycemia, seizures, and death. Diagnosis is made by measurement of 1-phosphofructoaldolase activity in a liver biopsy specimen. The suspicion should be based on a carefully obtained dietary and family history.

Incidence is estimated as 1 in 35,000 to 40,000 births.

### Tyrosinemia

In the workup of the infant or child with liver disease, an elevated level of the amino acid tyrosine is at times difficult to interpret. Nonspecific elevations can occur, regardless of the underlying etiology, and are often accompanied by an elevation of methionine concentrations as well. Tyrosinemia remains an elusive entity, and the diagnosis is always difficult, and fortunately, rare. Jaundice appears in the context of liver failure, which can occur at an early age. The liver shows advanced cirrhosis and the infant may present because of organomegaly and failure to thrive. Bone demineralization and ricketts result from a Fanconi renal tubular defect.

Special formulas low in tyrosine and phenylalanine should be given, and occasional case reports have documented improvement in liver and kidney function and a brighter prognosis. Care should be coordinated with a specialist in metabolic disorders, since monitoring of plasma amino acids is often useful during dietary management. Hepatomas are frequent complications in long lasting cases, and are indications for liver transplantation.

### Other Metabolic Disorders

Cholestatic jaundice can be an associated feature of several congenital syndromes involving the metabolism of bile acids (abnormal cholic acid synthesis, Zellweger's), lipids (Gaucher's, Neimann-Pick, Wolman's), and very rarely in cystic fibrosis, usually in association with inspissated bile plug syndrome rather than with the more typical lesions of biliary cirrhosis, which usually develops in later years.

## Anatomic

The main consideration in the investigation of a child with pale (acholic) stools and direct hyperbilirubinemia is to determine whether the obstruction requires surgical correction. The patient should be placed on phenobarbital in an attempt to stimulate the bile-acid independent bile flow, and studies should then be planned to image the liver and biliary tree. The most useful modalities include an abdominal ultrasonogram while the infant has been fasted for at least 5 hours, and an IDA scan after at least 5 days of phenobarbital stimulation. If possible, a nasoduodenal tube can be placed and samples of the drainage collected every hour for 18 or 24 hours. In conditions of intrahepatic cholestasis, some of the samples will show biliary pigments, ruling out complete obstruction of the biliary system. In experienced hands, this method has proven to be sensitive and specific. Unfortunately, few centers are presently enthusiastic about the intubations.

Ultrasonography will detect dilatation of the biliary tree, cystic abnormalities (both of the liver and the kidneys), and ascites. Choledochal cysts, spontaneous perforation of the bile ducts, and gallstones can also be diagnosed by an experienced examiner. In contrast with biliary obstruction in the adult, the intrahepatic ducts rarely show dilatation in the pediatric patient.

## BIBLIOGRAPHY

1. Maisels MJ: Jaundice in the newborn. *Pediatr Rev* 1982; 3:305.
2. Cockington RA: A guide to the use of phototherapy in the management of neonatal hyperbilirubinemia. *J Pediatr* 1979; 95:281.
3. Odievre M, Luzeau R: More on breast milk jaundice. *J Pediatr* 1982; 100:761.
4. Schmid R: Bilirubin: State of the art. *Gastroenterology* 1978; 74:1307.
5. Vaisman SL, Gartner LM: Pharmacologic treatment of neonatal hyperbilirubinemia. *Clin Perinatal* 1975; 2:37.
6. Danks CM, Campbell PE, Smith AL, et al: Prognosis of babies with neonatal hepatitis. *Arch Dis Child* 1977; 52:368.
7. Sinatra FR: Cholestasis in infancy and childhood: *Curr Probl Pediatr* 1982; 12:1–54.
8. Watson S, Giacoia GP: Cholestasis in infancy: A review. *Clin Pediatr* 1983; 22:30–36.

# 16

## Biliary Atresia

Biliary atresia refers to the obliteration of the extrahepatic bile ducts by a progressive, fibrosing, inflammatory reaction of unknown etiology. In most cases, the gallbladder and the cystic duct are also involved at the time of presentation, although in other cases, only portions of the common bile duct or the common hepatic duct show complete fibrosis.

Biliary atresia is not just a disease of the bile ducts, but rather a condition of global involvement of the intra- and extrahepatic bile ducts as well as the hepatocyte. Whether the hepatocellular changes are secondary to biliary stasis or reflect a concurrent effect of the basic underlying process causing biliary atresia is not clear. Unfortunately, what is clear is that even when adequate bile drainage is established by corrective surgery, the changes in the liver and eventual biliary cirrhosis can continue to develop in the majority of the patients.

### INCIDENCE AND ETIOLOGY

Biliary atresia has been reported to occur in 1 out of every 10,000 to 20,000 live births. Interestingly, some clustering of cases has occurred, suggesting exposure to a common infectious or toxic agent. Initially thought to be a developmental abnormality, biliary atresia has not been detected in premature infants or stillborns. This speaks against a defect of embryogenesis and more in favor of an acquired lesion. In addition, abnormalities of the pancreas and its ducts are not seen in biliary atresia, an expected occurrence since both structures derive from a common anlage of the foregut endoderm.

In the 1960s, Landing proposed the concept of *obstructive cholangiopathy*, which included idiopathic neonatal hepatitis and biliary atresia on both ends of a spectrum of disease involving the liver and the intra- and extrahepatic bile ducts to various degrees. In some cases, the inflammatory reaction is preferentially confined to the liver and its structures, while in others, progressive sclerosing of the extrahepatic ducts takes place. Reports of children with patent extrahepatic ducts demonstrated by intraoperative cholangiography were explored at a later day for persistent jaundice, only to find histologic and anatomic evidence of biliary atresia.

The possibility that an infection with reovirus type 3 is responsible for biliary atresia is being investigated intensively, following initial work that showed seroconversion in 70% of affected patients, as opposed to 9% controls. This virus has an affinity for biliary epithelium in weanling mice and produces a picture that histologically resembles human biliary atresia. Clinically, the infection is self-limited in the mice and so behaves very differently than in the human. More recent work in an immunodeficient mouse model suggests that the infection can become chronic (and eventually result in liver failure) if the animal is unable to clear the virus. Identification of viral particles in tissues obtained at the time of surgery in humans has been difficult and might require special staining techniques. Viral proteins can potentially become incorporated in the genome of the cells and their presence be detected only with specific DNA probes.

## HISTOLOGIC APPEARANCE

Despite the inherent sampling errors that occur during percutaneous needle biopsy of the liver, the information obtained by this relatively safe procedure is valuable. Even when the patient is less than three months of age, cirrhosis is often present at the time of the initial assessment. The core of tissue obtained during the biopsy will crumble or fragment when advanced scarring is present in the liver. In contrast, cirrhosis is rarely established at this young age in neonatal hepatitis or metabolic liver disease.

In less advanced cases, inflammation in and around the portal area is present in association with bile duct proliferation. Giant cell transformation is a nonspecific response of the human newborn liver to a variety of noxious agents, and can be found in neonatal hepatitis or in biliary atresia. Proliferation of the intrahepatic bile ducts is more suggestive of an extrahepatic obstruction, but a paucity of bile ducts is often seen in the biopsies, and it might take some time before proliferation can be appreciated. Repeat biopsies will, in most cases, show the evolution of the lesion.

The pathological changes in the extrahepatic tissues, including the gall-bladder, include thick fibrous tissue proliferation, with or without inflammatory cells. The epithelium of the bile ducts is, when present, disrupted and abnormal looking. In most cases, the obliteration involves the ducts close to the porta hepatitis, while in a minority, atresia or severe stenosis of only the distal common bile duct is present.

*Differential Diagnosis*

Children with biliary atresia tend to be slightly small for dates, but otherwise their perinatal course is unremarkable. Physiologic jaundice might be present and more prolonged, but the peak of the bilirubin elevation is not unusually high. Congenital anomalies are rare in biliary atresia, except when it is part of the *polysplenia syndrome*. In this condition, mirror-image asymmetry of the abdominal viscera is present, with associated abnormalities in the vascular supply to the right lung (eparterial), nonrotation of the intestine, and abnormal development of the spleen, which can be present as multiple small islands of splenic tissue scattered throughout the abdominal cavity. Cardiac defects are sometimes present, most frequently ventricular septal defects.

In contrast to *neonatal hepatitis*, which is the major differential consideration, skin rashes or lesions, splenomegaly, or lymphadenopathy are not present. The presence of a heart murmur, peculiar facial characteristics, and ocular abnormalities should suggest the possibility of *Alagille's syndrome*. The facies in Alagille's syndrome includes prominent, rounded forehead, hypertelorism, and a pointed chin. Many children with cholestatic conditions present with similar characteristics, and the specificity of the features has been questioned. More important is the observation that patients with the constellation of findings described in the syndrome tend to have a better clinical outlook than patients with the "nonsyndromic" form of *intrahepatic paucity of bile ducts*. Progressive destruction of intrahepatic bile ducts and ductules results in a range of pathological findings, all of which can be included under the general classification of *bile duct hypoplasia*. Specific entities, such as *alpha-1-antitrypsin deficiency*, have a very similar pathological appearance, which only reflects the limited range of response of the liver to a host of different noxious stimuli.

*Diagnostic Evaluation*

The pediatrician who makes the important distinction between direct and indirect hyperbilirubinemia at an early stage in his evaluation of the child with persistent jaundice or acholic stools has contributed his share to the care of this patient. The most common reason for delayed diagnosis is the tendency to be complacent about mild jaundice in an infant who is otherwise clinically fine. Perhaps there is also the tendency to spare the parents the anxiety associated with a suspicion of liver disease, but there is really no reason to postpone doing a bilirubin fractionation in any child with jaundice after the neonatal period. Even if the infant is breast fed, a simple examination can reassure the doctor that waiting is safe.

### Laboratory Examinations

Additional laboratory examinations obtained from the office are usually not necessary and should be deferred to the pediatric gastroenterologist to avoid duplication. Workup can be carried out in a matter of days in a center with the facilities to perform the imaging studies and a good pathologist to review the liver biopsy.

During the last decade, the search for a test that will unquestionably distinguish between complete obstruction of the extrahepatic ducts and other cholestatic conditions not requiring surgery has resulted in a proliferation of specialized measurements, none of which fulfill the desired goal. The main reason for this difficulty is that if the intrahepatic cholestasis is severe enough, the end result as viewed from excretory, biochemical, or imaging studies will be indistinguishable from complete extrahepatic atresia. The effect of cholestasis on certain lipid fractions (lipoprotein X) and on the ratio of monohydroxy and dihydroxy bile acids after administration of the bile acid binding resin Cholestyramine were explored with great expectations, but here again, the degree of overlap is too large to allow postponement of an exploratory laparotomy with confidence.

## NUCLEAR SCANNING

Separate collection of stools and urine for measurement of radioactivity after intravenous administration of iodinated rose bengal was popular in the 1960s, but is cumbersome, requires bladder catheterization in female infants, and can be totally uninterpretable if urine contaminates the stool specimens. Administration of iodine was necessary to minimize incorporation of the isotope in the infant's thyroid. Excretion of less than 10% of the injected dose over the 72-hour collection was a strong suggestion of extrahepatic obstruction. The rose bengal excretion test is not available anymore and has been replaced by a nonquantitative nuclear scanning that uses one of a family of imide compounds that are incorporated into the hepatocyte and excreted in the bile in a similar manner to bilirubin. The IDA scan is performed after at least 5 days of stimulation of bile flow with phenobarbital at therapeutic dosage (5 mg/kg per day in two doses). If no visualization of the intestine occurs in the first 6 hours after injection, a delayed image is obtained after 24 hours. Failure to detect contrast in the intestine in a child who has no evidence of metabolic or infectious liver disease constitutes an indication for exploratory laparotomy. If the biopsy is consistent with neonatal hepatitis and the infant is younger than 12 weeks, treatment with phenobarbital is continued and a reevaluation and biopsy are done 2 to 4 weeks later.

## SURGERY

During the exploratory laparotomy, a small transverse incision is made below the right costal margin. The anatomy is examined and, if a well-developed gallbladder is present, intraoperative cholangiogram is done after aspirating the contents of the gallbladder. Pale, thick mucus is sometimes present in cases of complete extrahepatic obstruction, and its presence is not an indication of patency of the common hepatic duct. Inspection of the liver helps determine the extent of cirrhosis, which is already present at this time in over half of the patients. If patent ducts are demonstrated, and contrast reaches the duodenum, a wedge biopsy of both lobes of the liver is taken and the operation is terminated. If an atretic gallbladder is recognized, and the fibrous remnants of the extrahepatic ducts are identified, the incision is enlarged and the surgeon proceeds with the Kasai operation.

## THE KASAI OPERATION

Pioneered by Morio Kasai in Japan over 20 years ago, the operation that bears his name is presently the only available therapy for biliary atresia, short of transplantation. Numerous modifications have evolved after the original portoenterostomy, but the basic principle remains the creation of a conduit from a segment of jejunum that is anastomosed to the porta hepatis (Fig 16–1). The fibrous cone of the atretic ducts is dissected high in the hilum of the porta and the jejunal portion of the Roux-en-Y is brought up, allowing bile to be diverted into the intestine. The reason this operation has a chance to succeed is that patent bile ducts are present under the surface of the liver and the extrahepatic atresia affects the larger ducts preferentially. The size of the ducts is measured in frozen sections taken at the time of the dissection, and this determination has some prognostic implications as far as the chances for bile drainage is concerned.

### Prognosis

Untreated, biliary atresia is uniformly fatal. Death occurs between 6 months and 4 years of age as a result of liver failure and the complications of portal hypertension. Experience with the Kasai portoenterostomy has changed the natural course of the disease, although biliary cirrhosis can progress despite a "successful" operation, i.e., after resumption of bile flow and clearance of the jaundice.

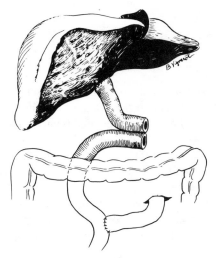

**FIG 16–1.**
Bilioenteric conduit constructed by John R. Lilly. The proximal (hepatic) aspect of the defunctionalized limb of the Roux-en-Y jejunostomy is exteriorized as a double-barreled jejunostomy. (From Welch KJ, Randolph JG, Ravitch MM, et al: *Pediatric Surgery*, ed. 4. Chicago, Year Book Medical Publishers, 1986. Used by permission.)

Follow-up studies of large numbers of patients operated on by experienced surgeons support an attitude of guarded optimism for at least one-third of the patients. Among these excellent results are children without any stigmata of chronic liver disease 5–8 years after their original operation. Usually, transaminase values remain permanently elevated. In another one-third of the patients, progressive cirrhosis develops in the ensuing years. Portal hypertension and variceal bleeding are frequent and, at least temporarily, amenable to sclerotherapy management. The appearance of ascites, hypoalbuminemia, coagulation abnormalities, and hypersplenism are signs of a poor prognosis and an indication for liver transplantation.

During the first 2 years of life, the most frequent complications include cholangitis and nutritional deficits. The diagnosis of cholangitis is often a clinical one, since positive blood cultures are the exception, and even liver tissue cultures obtained by percutaneous biopsies often fail to identify an organism. Enteric organisms, including anaerobes, are most often responsible for this complication, and broad spectrum intravenous antibiotics are needed to prevent the spread of the infection and the development of intrahepatic abscesses. Cholangitis tends to result in progressive scarring and in loss of parenchymal function.

Cholangitis should be suspected when the following signs and symptoms are present:

• Fever, sometimes spiking, without an apparent source

- Lethargy or irritability
- Anorexia
- Increased jaundice (scleral, darker urine)
- Acholic stools.

For reasons that are not clear, the incidence of cholangitis decreases after the first 2 years of life. Prompt hospitalization for antibiotic therapy is indicated at the first suspicion of cholangitis in the child with biliary atresia.

Because of the persistence of cholestasis in a large number of infants, absorption of dietary fat and of fat-soluble vitamins (A, D, E, and K) is suboptimal and requires attention to detail and close follow-up for adequate replacement.

Growth can be delayed despite supplements with MCT oil, and chronic malnutrition is a hallmark of severe liver disease. Simple carbohydrates and starches are better absorbed than fat-containing foodstuffs and can help improve total caloric intake. As a starting point, the following dosages of vitamins are recommended:

- Vitamin A: 10,000–20,000 IU/day
- Vitamin K: 5 mg once or twice a week
- Vitamin D: 5,000–10,000 IU/day $D_2$ or 3–5 µg/kg/day 25, hydroxycholecalciferol
- Vitamin E: 50–400 IU/kg/day.

The importance of normal vitamin E status has been clearly shown in both animal and human studies. Chronic deficiency results in a well-defined neurological syndrome presenting with loss of peripheral reflexes, ocular muscle paralysis, and retinal dysfunction. If detected before age 3 years and adequately treated (even if it requires intramuscular injections), the abnormalities can be prevented or improved. Longer-lasting deficits can be irreversible and permanent. When vitamin E status cannot be corrected even with the use of large doses of available "water soluble" preparations (150–200 IU/kg/day), the patient should be referred for treatment with an intramuscular formulation of dl-alpha-tocopherol (Ephynal; Hoffman-LaRoche, Inc.) or orally with a newly developed form of d-alpha-tocopheryl succinate suspended in polyethylene glycol-1000 (TPGS; Eastman Chemical Co.). At this time, both of these medications are only available through medical centers with special interest in childhood liver diseases.

## BIBLIOGRAPHY

1. Barkin RM, Lilly JR: Biliary atresia and the Kasai operation: Continuing care. *J Pediatr* 1980; 96:1915.
2. Devries P, Cox K: Surgical treatment of congenital and neonatal biliary obstruction. *Surg Clin North Am* 1981; 61:987.

3. Kasai M, Watanabi I, and Ryaji O: Follow-up studies of long term survivors after hepatic portoenterostomy for "non-correctable" biliary atresia. *J Pediatr Surg* 1975; 10173.
4. Altman RP, Levy J: Biliary atresia. *Pediatr Ann* 1985; 14:481–485.

# 17

## Infectious Hepatitis

In the last 10 years, it has become possible to diagnose hepatitis more accurately than ever before. Availability of serologic markers and development of new probes for the detection of specific IgM antibodies allows identification of a great variety of agents, and makes possible the distinction between recent and distant infection. Carrier states, need for prophylaxis, degree of infectivity, and epidemiologic questions can be answered with great certainty.

For the practitioner, once the diagnosis of hepatitis has been made on the basis of the biochemical abnormalities present, identification of the responsible agent becomes the obvious next step. Based on that information, the clinical course and prognosis can be predicted and proper measures taken to contain the disease in the household or in the community.

### CLINICAL FEATURES

Symptoms of hepatitis are nonspecific, and in a majority of cases, the inflammation is totally asymptomatic. Over 50% of cases are anicteric. There is little difference in the clinical presentations of symptomatic hepatitis according to its etiology, and for that reason diagnosis made on the basis of epidemiologic and circumstantial features is only tentative and needs confirmation by serological tests.

The spectrum of disease ranges from mild flu-like symptoms with low-grade temperature, malaise, anorexia, and minimal scleral icterus to such a fulminant disease that there is no time for great elevations in the bilirubin concentration. Encephalopathy and bleeding can evolve in a matter of hours or days. Hepatitis associated to Epstein-Barr virus infections can present in the context of clinical infectious mononucleosis or, more rarely, the liver can be the main target of the virus.

Less common presentations include the maculopapular, urticarial acrodermatitis of the *Gianotti-Crosti syndrome* and *glomerulitis* resulting in hematuria, oliguria, and edema. Personality changes associated with hepatitis include depression, lassitude, disinterest, and detachment.

Hepatitis due to cytomegalovirus, rubella, herpes, and toxoplasma are more common in the infant, usually as congenitally acquired infections. Coxsackie B virus can produce severe encephalitis and myocarditis, the liver being affected to various degrees, sometimes severely. Multisystem involvement is common. In the case of hepatitis A, B, delta, and non-A, non-B, the viruses are hepatotrophic and selectively attack the hepatocyte. Involvement of other systems (for example, joints, skin, and kidney) is often due to circulating immune complexes and not because of viral replication in those tissues.

## HEPATITIS A

After an average incubation period of 30 days (range 15 to 40 days), symptomatic hepatitis A presents acutely, with flu-like complaints, jaundice, low-grade fever, and tiredness (Fig 17–1). Diagnosis is straightforward, with a positive test for IgM anti-HA confirming acute infection. A negative IgM and positive IgG anti-HA indicates distant infection and natural immunity. Anicteric disease is more common in children than in adults (10:1). Its course also tends to be more severe in the adult.

The hepatitis A virus has an RNA genome and has been detected in feces of infected individuals 2 to 3 weeks before the onset of clinical disease. The period of viral shedding in the stool (and urine) is very short after the appearance of jaundice, a reason why extreme precautions are not necessary in the management of the family and contacts.

Epidemics with probable fecal-oral transmission are seen in conditions of poor hygiene and crowding and are endemic in many regions of the world, including the United States. Contaminated water has caused outbreaks in summer camps and other communities, frequently traced to raw seafood or contaminated fish. Parenteral transmission has also been shown to occur. The blood is infective during the period of incubation only.

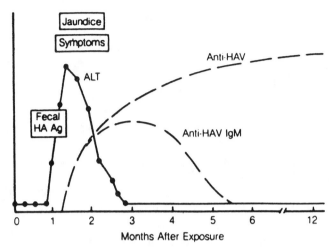

**FIG 17–1.**
The clinical, serological, and biochemical course of typical type A hepatitis. *HA Ag* = hepatitis A antigen; *ALT* = alanine aminotransferase; *Anti-HAV* = antibody to hepatitis A virus. (From Hoofnagle JH: *Perspectives on Viral Hepatitis.* North Chicago, Abbott Laboratories Diagnostic Division, 1981. Used by permission.)

## PROPHYLAXIS OF CONTACTS

Treatment of household contacts is indicated as soon as the diagnosis of acute hepatitis A is made and consists of intramuscular gamma globulin in a dose of 0.02–0.04 cc/kg body weight. Passive immunization modifies the clinical course of the illness but does not prevent acquisition of the infection. If the volume of gamma globulin is larger than 2 cc, the dose should be split in two and administered in both buttocks. As mentioned previously, no late sequelae of hepatitis A have been noted, but fulminant disease can occur in a small minority of cases (1 in 1,000), mainly adults. Immunity is lifelong.

## HEPATITIS B

A number of tests are available because of the multiplicity of antigens present in the Dane particle (Fig 17–2). This 42-nm particle represents the whole virion, and within its core is the double-stranded, incomplete, circular DNA with its associated DNA polymerase and other soluble proteins responsible for eliciting specific immunological responses.

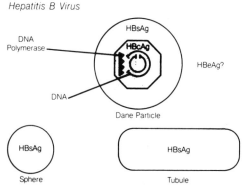

**FIG 17–2.**
Proposed structure of the hepatitis B virus. Note the incomplete double-stranded DNA in the virion and the presence of surface antigen in the envelope of the capsid. (From Hoofnagle JH: *Perspectives on Viral Hepatitis.* North Chicago, Abbott Laboratories Diagnostic Division, 1981. Used by permission.)

## SEROLOGIC MARKERS

The surface antigen *HBsAg* is the coating protein of the virion envelope and is the earliest serological *marker* to appear, sometimes 2–4 weeks before the aminotransferase elevations. The e antigen *HBeAg* has a brief rise shortly thereafter and disappears well before the HBsAg. Before the appearance of antibody to the surface antigen *anti-HBs*, there is a period during which the only *marker* present is the core antibody, *anti-HBc*. This "core window" occurs within 3 months of infection and lasts 2 to 16 weeks.

More recently it has become possible to detect specific antibodies to the core antigen in the IgM family of immunoglobulins. This *IgM anti-HBc* is good evidence of acute hepatitis B infection. When the patient has completely cleared the virus, only *anti-HBs, anti-HBc*, and *anti-HBe* are detectable (Fig 17–3). If there is no seroconversion and the patient becomes a carrier, HBsAg and anti-HBc are present, but no antibodies to the surface antigen are produced. If HBeAg is also detectable, high infectivity is present, more than 30,000 times the infectivity of serum positive only for HBsAg. HBeAg should not be checked unless HBsAg is positive since the yield of this test is nil in the absence of surface antigen. The clinical features are variable; the most common ones are malaise, anorexia, and nausea, which are sometimes prominent before jaundice becomes apparent (Fig 17–4).

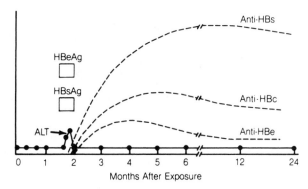

**FIG 17–3.**
Typical course of the major serological markers in acute hepatitis B infection.
(From Hoofnagle JH: *Perspectives on Viral Hepatitis.* North Chicago, Abbott Laboratories Diagnostic Division, 1981. Used by permission.)

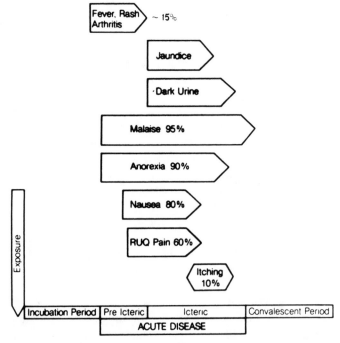

**FIG 17–4.**
Most common clinical features of acute hepatitis B and their relation to the icteric phase of the disease. (From Hoofnagle JH: *Perspectives on Viral Hepatitis.* North Chicago, Abbott Laboratories Diagnostic Division, 1981. Used by permission.)

# CHRONIC HEPATITIS B

One of the important features of hepatitis B infection is its propensity to become chronic in about 10% of cases. In comparison, non-A, non-B hepatitis can become chronic in 30%–45% of affected patients. No instance of chronic hepatitis A has been reported. Fulminant hepatitis can occur in 0.1% of all cases of hepatitis A and B. The risk is higher in children with immunodeficiencies.

The prevalence of the carrier state for hepatitis B virus is different in various parts of the world, being highest in the Far East where 5%–10% of the population harbor the virus in the hepatocytes. This accounts for the high incidence of hepatocellular carcinoma seen in the Chinese and South East Asian. Interestingly, the viral genome has been demonstrated in the DNA of the tumor cells and is even integrated in the DNA of normal appearing hepatocytes. Hopefully, with widespread immunization programs against hepatitis B infection, the epidemiology of these neoplasms will be radically affected.

The *carrier state* in the American population has been estimated at 0.1%– 0.2% but is much higher in selected populations such as health professionals, hemophiliacs, renal dialysis patients and personnel, dentists, intravenous drug addicts, and homosexuals.

The carrier state is defined by the presence of surface antigen (with or without e antigen) for over 6 months and a failure to develop anti-HBs. Occasionally, a *late seroconversion* will take place in someone previously labelled a chronic carrier. Asymptomatic carriers may or may not have biochemical evidence of hepatitis, but it is becoming clear that even in the absence of abnormal aminotransferase elevations, chronic and progressive damage to the liver can take place.

When the transaminases have been abnormal for more than 6 months, the distinction between *chronic active* and *chronic persistent hepatitis* needs to be considered, mainly for prognostic purposes. A liver biopsy is necessary to make that distinction, and the presence of associated cirrhosis and piecemeal necrosis implies accelerated damage to the liver and an estimated 5-year survival of 50%, while chronic persistent hepatitis is much less aggressive and carries a brighter prognosis (95%–98% 5-year survival).

## Perinatal Transmission of Hepatitis B Infection

An important contribution to the management of infants born to HBsAg+ mothers is the availability of hyperimmune gamma globulin with high titers against hepatitis B virus (HBIG) and the possibility of eliciting the infant's own immune response with a *hepatitis B vaccine*. Recognition of the infant at risk is crucial. Mothers from geographic areas of high endemicity should be screened for their serologic status to hepatitis B as part of prenatal care. Routine evaluation of *all* pregnant mothers has been recommended by some in view of the high degree of infant infection and risk of chronic hepatitis.

Administration of HBIG (0.5 cc IM) is done in the delivery room, and the first dose of vaccine is given within 24 hours (0.5 cc IM in the arm) and then a booster at 3 months.

Although mothers who are e antigen positive and those who contract hepatitis in the last trimester are more infectious, prophylactic treatment should be given to all infants born to HBsAg+ mothers, regardless of their e antigen status. Immunization (passive and active) does not require withholding of breast feedings. Chronic B antigenemia is thus effectively prevented in this population and the occurrence of hepatitis B (fulminant and chronic) almost completely avoided.

Presently, the use of hepatitis B vaccine is also recommended in:

• Patients and staff in renal dialysis units
• Immunosuppressed patients
• Household contacts of hepatitis BsAg carriers
  (In addition, infants and older children should also receive HBIG)
• Individuals admitted or working in institutions at high risk
• Homosexuals, individuals with multiple sex partners, intravenous drug users
• All health care personnel exposed to patients' secretions or blood.


## NON-A, NON-B HEPATITIS (NANB)

The diagnosis of NANB hepatitis remains one of exclusion. Most transfusion-related hepatitis is NANB since the institution of widespread screening of donors. Clinically, the disease is indistinguishable from A or B hepatitis, although it tends to be somewhat less severe than the latter and the aminotransferase elevations are less prominent. The duration of the biochemical abnormalities tends to parallel the course in hepatitis A (i.e., less than 4 weeks).

A fulminant course and chronic hepatitis are the two more worrisome aspects of this infection and reflect deranged immune responses on the part of the host. Identification of the agent(s) responsible and development of serologic markers will allow positive diagnosis of these infection(s) and shed light on their epidemiology, clinical course, and outcome.


## DELTA HEPATITIS

The delta agent is an incomplete RNA virus that can only exist in the presence of the hepatitis B virus since it uses the synthetic apparatus of this virus for its own replication.

TABLE 17–1.
Summary of Suggested Evaluations

1. To diagnose Hepatitis A:
   IgM and IgG anti-HA
2. To diagnose acute Hepatitis B:
   HBsAg. If positive:
   HBeAg and anti-HBe
   Also, if available:
   IgM anti-HBc
3. To decide on the need for HBIG prophylaxis in cases of parenteral exposure:
   Check HBsAg in the person causing the exposure. If negative, no need for HBIG in the exposed person.
   Check anti-HBs in the person exposed. If positive, no need for HBIG.
4. For assessment of infectivity in HBsAg+ individual:
   HBeAg and anti-HBe
5. For assessment of anti-HBc + chronic active hepatitis patient:
   anti-HD. If possible, also IGM anti-HD to differentiate between chronic delta infection or recent superinfection.

The importance of the delta agent is its involvement in the more severe forms of B hepatitis, both fulminant and chronic. Infection occurs parenterally, either coincidentally with B infection ("coinfection") or superimposed with it in a chronic carrier ("superinfection").

Progress in the elucidation of the biology of delta hepatitis has been rapid since the agent was identified in the livers of patients with fulminant hepatitis in the 1970s and in a devastating epidemic outbreak among the Yupca Indians in Venezuela. Anti-HD antibodies can now be measured by radioimmunoassay in several commercial laboratories, and further refinements allow detection of ongoing infection by specific IgM-anti-HD antibodies. In addition, monoclonal immune staining permits demonstration of the delta virus in liver biopsy material.

Delta hepatitis seems to be more common in certain geographic areas, for example, Italy, South America, and the Pacific United States. Its epidemiology also correlates with that of chronic B hepatitis, particularly when it is HBeAg + .

Chronic delta hepatitis has a tendency to evolve into cirrhosis and contributes to increased morbidity and mortality. Interestingly, batches of immunoglobulins prepared as far back as 1940 have titers against the delta agent, suggesting that this incomplete virus has been involved in human disease for much longer than was initially recognized.

A summary of suggested evaluations in the investigation of the patient with suspected hepatitis is presented in Table 17–1. The interpretation of hepatitis A, B serologic markers appears in Table 17–2.

TABLE 17–2.
Summary of Interpretation of Serological Tests

| | |
|---|---|
| 1. HBsAg −, anti-HBs −, anti-HBc − | Hepatitis B unlikely |
| 2. HBsAg +, anti-HBs −, anti-HBc − | Acute HB infection if available, confirm with IgM anti-HBc |
| 3. HBsAg +, anti-HBs −, anti-HBc + | Acute HB infection or carrier |
|    If, in addition HBeAg + and anti-HBe − | High infectivity present |
|    If available, obtain anti-delta antibodies | |
| 4. HBsAg −, anti-HBs −, anti-HBc + | Persistent HB infection; also, early HB convalescence |
| 5. HBsAg −, anti-HBs +, anti-HBc − or + | Immune to HB virus |
| 6. Anti-HA IgM −, anti-HA IgG − | Hepatitis A unlikely |
| 7. Anti-HA IgM +, anti-HA IgG − | Acute hepatitis A (4–6 weeks) |
| 8. Anti-HA IgM −, anti-HA IgG + | Immune to hepatitis A |

# BIBLIOGRAPHY

1. DelaPlane D, Yogev R, Crussi F, et al: Fatal hepatitis B in early infancy: The importance of identifying HBsAg-positive in pregnant women and providing immunoprophylaxis to their newborns. *Pediatrics* 1983; 72:176–180.
2. Hadler VC, Webster HM, Erber JJ, et al: Hepatitis A in day care centers: A community-wide assessment. *N Engl J Med* 1980; 302:1222.
3. Beasley RP, Hwang LY, Stevens CE, et al: Efficacy of hepatitis B immune globulin for prevention of perinatal transmission of the hepatitis B virus carrier state: Final report of a randomized double-blind, placebo-controlled trial. *Hepatology* 1983; 3:135–151.
4. Krugman S: Viral hepatitis B: Studies in natural history and prevention re-examined. *N Engl J Med* 1979; 30:101.
5. Nishioka NS, Dienstag JL: Delta hepatitis: A new scourge? (Editorial). *N Engl J Med* 1985; 312(23):1515–1516.
6. Perrilo RP: Differentiation between recent and remote hepatitis infections. *J Intern Med* 1984; (6):123–142.
7. Gimson AES, White YS, Eddelston ALW, et al: Clinical and prognostic differences in fulminant hepatitis type A, B, and non-A non-B. *Gut* 1983; 24:1194–1198.
8. Moestrup T, Hansonn BG, Widell A, et al: Clinical aspects of delta infection. *Br Med J* 1983; 286:87–90.
9. Farci P, Smedile A, Lavarini C, et al: Delta hepatitis in inapparent carriers of hepatitis B surface antigen. *Gastroenterology* 1983; 85:669–673.

# 18

## Chronic Liver Disease

The management of the child with chronic liver disease will often be a partnership between the primary practitioner and the specialist. Guidance provided after the initial evaluation helps delineate follow-up plans and is useful in maintaining continuity of care, so important for the well-being of the child and family.

If the specialist is located in a distant referral center, the primary physician will be the one to assess the child regularly and will be responsible for identifying and evaluating findings pertinent to the status and progression of the liver condition. For this reason, familiarity with the more common chronic liver disorders and the impact of compromised liver function on physiological homeostasis is crucial.

Pharmacological and nutritional intervention to control ascites, prevent vitamin deficiencies, and maintain anti-inflammatory regimens (steroids, immunosuppressants) are some of the important aspects of the long-term care of these patients.

### CIRRHOSIS

Chronic liver disease, whether secondary to a metabolic inborn error of metabolism, a postinfectious sequelae, or a result of prolonged bile duct obstruction, often results in cirrhosis.

The histologic hallmarks of this condition are increased liver fibrosis, collapse of the normal lobule architecture, and the formation of regenerative nodules, (islands of hepatocytes surrounded by dense connective tissue). The percutaneous biopsy might underestimate the degree of scarring because it is difficult to aspirate representative tissue. A wedge biopsy obtained at laparoscopy or by minilaparotomy is more informative.

## PORTAL HYPERTENSION

The hemodynamic effects of portal vein encroachment by fibrosis is the development of portal hypertension and the formation of intra- and extrahepatic portosystemic anatomoses (Fig 18–1). The shunting of splanchnic blood away from the liver into collateral channels off the caval system is responsible for many of the complications experienced by the patient after long-lasting cirrhosis. Portal hypertension can also result from a prehepatic portal block (such as is seen in congenital hepatic fibrosis or portal vein thrombosis), with essentially normal parenchymal liver cell function. The prognosis of portal hypertension in this condition is more favorable and responds well to shunting operations.

Increased venous flow and engorgement of the submucosal esophageal and gastric veins is responsible for the development of esophageal varices. Variceal bleeding is a serious complication of portal hypertension.

The most common sign of portal hypertension is the presence of splenomegaly. Normally, the spleen is not a palpable organ in children. A spleen tip is not uncommonly found in young infants or when lung overinflation flattens the diaphragm. During intercurrent infections, Kuppfer cell hyperplasia sometimes enlarges the spleen and makes it detectable on physical examination. Generalized lymphadenopathy is likely to be present then.

Other signs of portal hypertension are periumbilical collaterals ("caput medusa"), only present when the block is intrahepatic, and more rarely, rectal shunts engorging the superior hemorrhoidal veins.

The risk of bleeding from esophageal varices increases with the duration of portal hypertension and with deterioration of liver function. On rare occasions, spontaneous decompression (usually temporary) can take place between the splenic and left renal veins providing a path away from the submucosal plexus.

Since the advent of neonatal intensive care and the common use of umbilical vein catheterization, prehepatic portal hypertension has occurred as a result of thrombosis of the portal vein or its branches and the development of *cavernous transformation*. Occlusion and partial recanalization of the portal vein seem to be the result of trauma to the intima or of injury due to the hypertonicity of the solutions infused. Cavernous transformation can also be idiopathic, often presenting with other associated anomalies, mainly cardiovascular. A history of

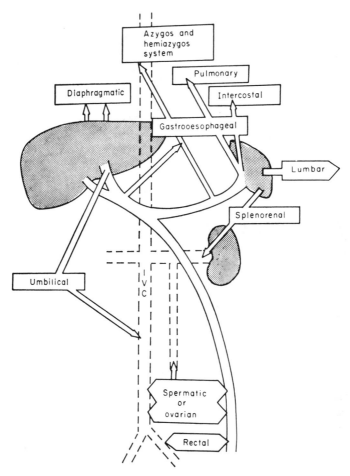

**FIG 18–1.**
Schematic representation of the most important portosystemic anastomoses that develop during the course of portal hypertension. (From Sherlock S: *Diseases of the Liver and Biliary Systems*, ed 6. Boston, Blackwell Scientific Publications, 1981. Used by permission.)

umbilical vein catheterization or omphalitis should be sought when evaluating any child with unexplained splenomegaly.

## ASCITES

A combination of factors contribute to the formation of ascites, the accumulation of fluid in the peritoneal cavity, including (1) intrahepatic capillary and lymphatic congestion and (2) decreased oncotic pressure secondary to hypoproteininemia and hypoalbuminemia, both of which favor exudation of fluid from the liver. Additional factors to be considered are expanded plasma volume and hyperaldosteronism from the abnormal hormone metabolism by decreased hepatocellular function. Avid salt retention by the kidneys contributes to increased total body water and worsens ascites.

## Management of Portal Hypertension and Ascites

Massive enlargement of the spleen results in hypersplenism. Neutropenia is usually not accompanied by the same propensity to infection seen in a similar reduction of the white count due to bone marrow failure.

Decreased phagocytic reserve can result in spontaneous peritonitis or infected ascites. More serious problems are caused by the progressive thrombocytopenia. The risk of bleeding significantly increases with the coagulopathy from the underlying liver disease.

The management of life-threatening splenomegaly includes portosystemic shunting (which tends to worsen hepatic function) and more recently, selective splenic artery embolization. The latter procedure must be done over a period of weeks, with intravenous antibiotic coverage. Splenic abscess is a complication, but results from experienced centers have been encouraging. In addition, decreased arterial flow to the spleen results in a decrease in portal flow with improvement of portal hypertension, at least temporarily. Ascites can develop insidiously or might appear suddenly, especially after a variceal bleed or recurrent bouts of cholangitis.

Initial measures to control fluid accumulation include a low-sodium diet (1–2 mEq/kg/day or 23–46 mg/kg/day) and spironolactone, 2.5–5 mg/kg/day in two divided doses. Spironolactone has potassium-sparing effects and is particularly appropriate because of its aldosterone inhibition. Potassium intake should be generous (3–4 mEq/kg/day) and electrolyte monitoring needs to be done regularly. After 5 days, if no improvement is noted (weight, girth), the spironolactone dosage can be increased and a thiazide diuretic added to the regimen (chlorothiazide, 5–10 mg/kg day).

An important warning to give to the parents is the complete avoidance of aspirin and aspirin-containing products, mainly cold medications. Acetaminophen can, in most cases, be safely administered even to the child with advanced cirrhosis. Parents should also be familiar with the signs and symptoms of variceal bleed and be given instructions to effectively handle the situation when it occurs. An up-to-date medical summary is useful to emergency room personnel and saves a lot of confusion during those stressful times. Fortunately, the first variceal bleed is usually well tolerated, especially in the patient with extrahepatic portal hypertension.

# BIBLIOGRAPHY

1. Schaffner F: Management of chronic hepatitis. *Semin Liver Disease* 1984; 5(3):209–219.
2. Alagille D: Management of chronic cholestasis in childhood. *Semin Liver Dis* 1984; 5(3):254–262.
3. Starzl TE, Iwatsuki S, Shaw BW, et al: Analysis of liver transplantation. *Hepatology* 1984; 4:47–49.
4. Wyllie R, Arasu TS, Fitzgerald JF: Ascites: Pathophysiology and management. *J Pediatr* 1980; 97:167.
5. Rogers EL, Rogers MC: Fulminant hepatic failure and hepatic encephalopathy. *Pediatr Clin North Am* 1980; 27:702.

# 19

# Biliary Tract Disease

Increased awareness of the involvement of the gallbladder in disease processes in infants and older children has been the direct result of the widespread use of ultrasonography. Advances in the identification of accurate anatomical localization of biliary tract obstruction, extent of involvement, and associated anomalies in the pancreas have helped greatly in our approach to some of the most challenging and demanding areas of the gastrointestinal tract. In the process, the management of "silent" gallstones has become a controversial issue since the natural history of such stones is poorly understood.

Congential abnormalities in the gallbladder and biliary tree can appear in infancy or be quiescent until adolescence or adulthood. Symptoms are a result of obstruction and infection. *Hydrops of the gallbladder* refers to the distention of the gallbladder in the absence of infection or mechanical block by stones. It is not as common as an isolated problem but occurs in association with other intercurrent illnesses, mainly sepsis, mucocutaneous lymph node syndrome (Kawasaki's disease), or in the presence of abnormalities of the cystic duct.

The most important malformations involve the biliary tree and the gallbladder to various extents, termed *choledochal cysts*. The cystic dilatations can be limited to the common bile duct or extend to one or both hepatic ducts (Fig 19–1). Abnormalities of the insertion of the pancreatic duct, duplication of the gallbladder, maldevelopment of the epithelial lining of the biliary tree, and secondary

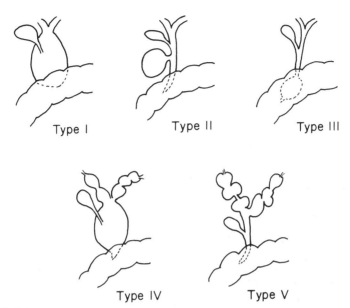

**FIG 19–1.**
Classification of choledochal cysts according to cholangiographic appearance. (From Welch KJ, Randolph JG, Ravitch MM, et al:*Pediatric Surgery*, ed 4. Chicago, Year Book Medical Publishers, 1986. Used by permission.)

changes in the liver compatible with biliary cirrhosis are sometimes prominent aspects of the clinical picture.

Symptoms of choledochal cysts can be vague and diagnosis is sometimes delayed until adolescence. In the infant, symptoms and signs are those of obstructive jaundice as described in Chapter 16. Recurrent abdominal pains can be gathered from the history, but in retrospect, they are often followed by long asymptomatic periods. Intermittent jaundice or change in urine color can be elicited in one third of the patients. Incidence of choledochal cysts is four times higher in Orientals, and they are more common in females for unclear reasons. The differential diagnosis includes acute cholecystitis, acute appendicitis, pancreatitis (which in fact can be an associated complication secondary to abnormal insertion and drainage of the pancreatic duct), or ectopic pregnancy.

The classic triad of a right upper quadrant mass, pain, and jaundice is found in less than 20% of patients. Diagnosis is usually made by ultrasonography, but for further anatomical definition, the surgeon will benefit from direct imaging of the biliary and pancreatic ducts. This is accomplished with percutaneous transhepatic cholangiography or with endoscopic retrograde choledochopancreatography. The cysts are treated surgically, and progressive hepatic damage can be avoided with early release of the obstruction. The recommended operation is excision of the cysts and creation of a new biliary conduit with construction of a Roux-en-Y from the gallbladder or the normal bile duct to the jejunum.

*Segmental dilatations of the biliary tree* can be isolated findings in the extra- and intrahepatic ducts and probably result from poor development of the muscular layer of those ducts. Symptoms are similar to those described for choledochal cysts. Therapy is surgical. Congenital dilatation of the intrahepatic bile ducts, also called *Caroli's disease,* is inherited as an autosomal recessive trait and has been reported mainly in males. The larger bile ducts show dilatations. Bile stasis can be marked, resulting in recurrent bouts of cholangitis. Symptoms include sepsis (sometimes fatal), bacteremia, right upper quadrant tenderness, and in- termittent, mild jaundice. Because of the associated impairment with bile salt excretion, fat and fat-soluble vitamin malabsorption can be present and the hepatic source of the problem considered in the investigations.

*Congenital duplication cysts* of the ducts and/or the gallbladder, *abnormal insertion of abnormal or aberrant bile ducts,* and *absence of the gallbladder* have also been described in infants and older patients. It is important to keep these variants in mind when considering surgical management of abnormalities in the biliary tree and gallbladder.

## GALLSTONES

Mechanisms of gallstone formation reflect the interaction between bile compo- nents, gallbladder dynamics, and triggers of nidus formation such as infection. The role of gallbladder contractility (or lack thereof) as seen in long periods of fasting or during the use of intravenous alimentation appears to be an important contributing factor to the formation of stones. Gallbladder atony occurs during pregnancy, a particularly high-risk time for gallstone formation. The composition of bile is a delicate balance of cholesterol, bile salts, and phospholipids. Dis- proportionate changes among these components can favor supersaturation of bile with cholesterol and cause precipitation around a nidus. The characteristics of gallbladder mucus and the physiology of fluid and electrolyte reabsorption and secretion are additional candidate factors in the etiology of cholelithiasis.

Gallstones can occur at any age, including the newborn period. Associated clinical features in this group can include neonatal sepsis, hypoxia, use of di- uretics, and anomalies in the gallbladder, bile ducts, and pancreas. In older children it may be associated with terminal ileal disease (such as in Crohn's disease or surgical resection) with loss and depletion of the bile acid pool. Chronic steatorrhea, as seen in cystic fibrosis, can change the composition of bile in a similar manner and helps explain the higher incidence in these patients. He- molytic anemias (hemoglobinopathies, spherocytosis, Wilson's disease) are well known predisposing factors for bilirubin stone formation.

## Symptoms

Recurrent abdominal pain is the most common symptom. It tends to occur in the right upper quadrant or epigastric area, and typically radiates to the shoulder and back. Anorexia, fat intolerance, and vomiting can be present in 50% of the patients. If cholecystitis is present, the clinical picture will be consistent with an intra-abdominal infection, sometimes with extreme prostration and toxicity and peritoneal signs, and the laboratory tests will confirm suppurative inflammation.

## Diagnosis

The most useful tests to document the presence of gallstones and associated gallbladder disease are the ultrasonogram and the IDA scan. The sonogram visualizes stones whether calcified or not. Thickening of the wall is a nonspecific finding, and the implications of detecting "sludge" are not totally clear, except to suggest bile stasis and poor gallbladder dynamics. The failure to visualize the gallbladder after the intravenous injection of $^{99m}$Tc-IDA tracer has been found to correlate with cystic duct obstruction/spasm in the presence of stone and cholecystitis. A normal oral cholecystogram and negative ultrasound of the gall-bladder rule out gallstones with 98% to 99% certainty. Important additional tests include a serum amylase, liver functions, complete blood count, and sedimentation rate. Blood cultures, chest x-rays, and scout film of the abdomen will help clarify important points in the differential diagnosis and will determine whether the stones are calcified or not.

## Treatment

For the patient with gallstones that result in clear-cut symptoms (obstruction, cholecystitis, pancreatitis, recurrent pains), surgery is curative. Exploration of the common bile duct might also be indicated if retained stones are suspected. Dissolution of cholesterol stones with chenodeoxycholate or ursodeoxycholate and newer percutaneous approaches with chemical dissolution of pigment stones is being tried in adults, but application of those techniques and approaches to the pediatric patient await further experience and definition of the ideal candidates.

# BIBLIOGRAPHY

1. Lau GE, Andrassy RJ, Hossein MG: A 30 year review of the management of gall-bladder disease at a children's hospital. *Am Surg* 1983; 49:411–413.
2. Buschi AJ, Brenbridge A: Sonographic diagnosis of cholelithiasis in childhood. *Am J Dis Child* 1980; 134:575.
3. Cooperberg PL, Burhenne HJ: Real-time ultrasonography: Diagnostic technique of choice in calculous gallbladder disease. *N Engl J Med* 1980; 302:1277–1279.
4. Babbitt DP, Starshak RJ, Clementt AR: Choledochal cyst: A concept of etiology. *AJR* 1973; 119:57–62.
5. Case 6–1977. *N Engl J Med* 1977; 296:328–335.
6. Tchirkow G, Highman LM, Shafer AD: Cholelithiasis and cholecystitis in children after repair of congenital duodenal anomalies. *Arch Surg* 1980; 115:85–86.

# Index